HEALTHY CROCKERY COOKERY

Books by Mable Hoffman

Mable Hoffman's Crockery Cookery
Healthy Crockery Cookery
Pot Luck

Most HPBooks are available at special quantity discounts for bulk purchases for sales promotions, premiums, fund-raising or educational use. Special books, or book excerpts, can also be created to fit specific needs.

For details, write: Special Markets, The Berkley Publishing Group, 375 Hudson Street, New York, New York 10014.

HEALTHY CROCKERY COOKERY

※

Mable Hoffman

HPBOOKS

HPBooks
Published by The Berkley Publishing Group
A division of Penguin Putnam Inc.
375 Hudson Street
New York, New York 10014

Copyright © 1998 by Mable Hoffman
Book design by Oksana Kusnir
Cover design by Charles Björklund
Cover photography by Zeva Oelbaum (Spinach and Prosciutto
Turkey Roulades, page 72, and Summer Vegetable Medley, page 171)
Interior photography by Glenn Cormier/Cormier Photography
Food Stylist: David Pogul

First edition: May 1998

Published simultaneously in Canada.

The Penguin Putnam Inc. World Wide Web site address is
http://www.penguinputnam.com

Library of Congress Cataloging-in-Publication Data
Hoffman, Mable.
Healthy crockery cookery / Mable Hoffman. — 1st ed.
        p.   cm.
Includes index.
ISBN 1-55788-290-8
1. Electric cookery, Slow.   2. Casserole cookery.   I. Title.
TX827.H5694   1998
    641.5′884—dc21   97–38976
                CIP

Printed in the United States of America
15   14   13

CONTENTS

Acknowledgments   vii

Introduction   1

Feast on Soups and Chili   9

Around the World with Chicken   35

Slow-Cooking Turkey Discoveries   67

Welcome Ways with Beef   91

Satisfying Tastes with Pork and Lamb   117

Good Eating with Wraps and Sandwiches   137

Slow-and-Easy Beans and Grains   149

From the Garden to the Slow Cooker   167

Year-Round Desserts and Accompaniments   185

Metric Conversion Charts   204

Index   205

ACKNOWLEDGMENTS

Special thanks to Jan Robertson for her invaluable assistance. Thanks to Grace Wheeler for recipe testing and to Mike Robertson for word processing.

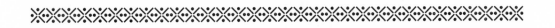

INTRODUCTION

Healthful Cooking in the Slow Cooker

*F*oods prepared in slow cookers yield healthful yet hearty meals. This is due to the slow, moist cooking method and to starting with the right ingredients. By using a slow cooker, the natural juices from meats and vegetables are retained in the pot rather than boiled away, resulting in flavorful, juicy, and nutritious dishes.

Most of our main dishes start with lean meats or poultry, which are enhanced with herbs or spices. They are cooked with popular vegetables that contribute moisture and flavor as well as important vitamins and minerals.

In this book, we have emphasized the healthy advantages of slow cooking for family meals without imposing drastic dietary limitations. We have included foods that children and teenagers enjoy and that families like to eat together, while maintaining a healthy balance with limited fat.

Because the slow cooker does not need fat for cooking there is little added fat except in the case of some desserts. Fat content of the recipes is controlled by choosing lean meats and trimming off the fat before cooking and by removing excess fat, and often the skin, from poultry.

Here are a few of the guidelines we followed in developing the recipes for this book.

- When purchasing meat, look for the leaner cuts.
- For cuts of meat with visible strips of fat around the edges, carefully trim off and discard the fat before placing the meat in the slow cooker.
- Although a small amount of marbling is flavorful in a pot roast, you can reduce the fat content by first browning both sides of the roast in a regular skillet. Then add the browned pot roast to the slow cooker with the seasonings and vegetables.
- Slightly reduce the size of meat servings. Currently the recommended amount per serving is about 3 ounces of cooked meat.
- Increase the proportion of vegetables in any slow cooker recipe that includes meats and vegetables.
- To extend meat or chicken flavor in soups or stews

without excess fat or calories, add a can of beef broth or fat-free chicken broth.

- If the cut of meat has more fat than you would like, make your slow cooker dish the day before you plan to use it. Transfer the dish to a bowl, refrigerate it overnight, and skim off the hard fat on the surface before reheating the dish. This technique works particularly well with soups and stews.
- Cook any large cut of meat on a rack in the slow cooker. Discard cooking juices, skim off surface fat, or only use a small amount of the fat-laden juices to cut the calories and fat content.

Using a Slow Cooker

The traditional slow cooker is a small electric appliance with a heating unit in the bottom. Basically, it is made with a crockery-lined container in which the food is actually cooked. Most of today's pots have a removable liner, but many of the older units had liners that were not removable. Both models may be used successfully, but the removable lining is more convenient and practical for serving food and cleanup.

The slow cookers are well insulated to ensure even cooking with an automatic control for a predetermined temperature. The cook can count on today's slow cookers to remain at the correct temperature. This feature enables the cook to enjoy a game of golf with friends, attend a teacher's conference, or spend a day at the office with the knowledge that dinner will be ready and waiting upon returning home.

Low or High?

Controls are usually limited to LOW, HIGH, and OFF. For traditional slow cooking as indicated in most of these recipes, the LOW setting is used. This enables the food to cook for a longer time, thereby retaining more vitamins and flavor. There's no worry about food drying out or burning on the bottom. You can put your favorite recipe in the slow cooker, cover it, plug it in, and let it cook on LOW for several hours while you engage in your favorite activities. If you are running a little late arriving home, the food will still be okay.

To Stir or Not to Stir

Usually, it is not necessary to stir foods while they are cooking in a crockery-lined pot. The exception to this is some of the dried-bean dishes.

When to Cook on High

We have indicated when to use the HIGH control in the directions for a few individual recipes. Although dried beans may be cooked on LOW, it takes so many hours that it would be impractical for most families. Thus we suggest using the HIGH control for dried-bean dishes. Each recipe specifies a length of time appropriate for that combination of ingredients.

Often vegetables such as mature carrots, rutabagas, parsnips, and other root vegetables take extra time in a slow cooker that is set on LOW. If you are pressed for time and the vegetables aren't done, turn the control to HIGH to speed up the cooking process. Another tip for cooking root vegetables: Arrange root vegetables on the bottom of the slow cooker and top with sauce or other ingredients for more even cooking.

We have found that making gravy or thickened sauce is more successful if you remove large pieces of meat after they are done. First set the meat aside and cover it loosely with foil to keep it warm. Then turn the slow cooker to HIGH and stir dissolved flour or cornstarch into the pan juices. Cook on HIGH for a few minutes. The actual length of time will depend on the amount of liquid in the pot. You may want to stir the mixture occasionally for a smoother sauce. For smaller pieces of meat, such as stew, leave the cooked meat in the pot and follow the same procedure.

Why Use a Slow Cooker?

Slow cookers fit into the life-style of today's family. With more people spending time away from home, this method enables busy parents to cook nourishing food without having to keep watch, while family members are busy at work, school, or recreation. Because many of the dishes require only a salad or perhaps a whole-grain bread to form a complete meal, the meal can be assembled quickly.

The slow cooker is also perfect for serving dishes on a buffet and for taking a dish to a potluck dinner.

Nutritional Analysis

All recipes were analyzed using a nutritional database. If the recipe lists a range for ingredients or number of servings, the smaller amount is used. Optional ingredients are not included in the analysis.

Percentage of Fat in the Diet

The recommended percentage of calories from fat is 30 percent as the average for the total diet. Some foods and even some meals in a healthy diet may exceed this amount without causing concern. What is important is that the average diet is around the recommended level of fat. As you plan meals, balance higher-fat foods with low-fat or non-fat choices.

For instance, someone eating 2,000 calories a day should consume about 65 grams total of fat. Only about 10 percent or less of the total fat should be from saturated fat.

Reducing Sodium

To further reduce the amounts of sodium used in these recipes, substitute reduced- or low-sodium products for the regular bouillon granules, broths, soy sauce, and canned items. For example, reduced-sodium bouillon granules have one-third less sodium than the regular granules. Draining and rinsing canned dried beans will reduce their sodium content.

If you need to reduce sodium intake for health reasons, always read the nutritional labels to determine the sodium content before purchasing items such as canned goods, prepared sauces, and ready-to-eat foods.

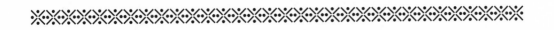

FEAST ON SOUPS AND CHILI

What is more appetizing after a tough day at the office than the aromatic flavors of a pot of soup or chili greeting you when you open your front door? There's no worry about overcooking or burning if you are away from home slightly longer than expected.

Slow cookers seem to maximize flavors, using only a minimum amount of meat. In many recipes, we have extended meat or chicken flavors with the addition of broth or bouillon. We have found that fat-free canned chicken broth is especially handy for this purpose. Turkey sausage or small amounts of well-trimmed lean meats also provide meaty flavors with very little fat.

✳ FRAGRANT BROWN RICE AND MUSHROOM SOUP

*A*n array of spices adds an exotic flavor to this soup—an ideal starter or an entree when served with a salad.

MAKES 8 TO 10 SERVINGS

3/4 cup long-grain brown rice

6 ounces mushrooms, finely chopped (about 2 cups)

1 medium onion, finely chopped

1 large stalk celery, finely chopped

1 teaspoon ground mustard

1 teaspoon ground black pepper

1/2 teaspoon salt

1/4 teaspoon ground coriander

1/8 teaspoon ground cardamom

1/8 teaspoon ground cinnamon

1/8 teaspoon ground cloves

6 cups beef bouillon or stock

1/3 cup chopped fresh cilantro leaves

1/4 cup nonfat plain yogurt

3 tablespoons finely chopped green onions, including some tops

Combine all ingredients, except cilantro leaves, yogurt, and green onions in a 3 1/2-quart slow cooker. Cover and cook on LOW 5 to 6 hours or until rice is tender. Stir in chopped cilantro. Ladle into soup bowls and garnish each serving with a dollop of yogurt and chopped green onion.

Per serving: Cal 92 · Carb 16 gm · Prot 5 gm · Total fat 1 gm · Sat fat 0 gm · Cal from fat 9 · Chol 0 mg · Sodium 733 mg

ROASTED RED PEPPER AND EGGPLANT SOUP

*T*his peasant-type soup is delicious with either shredded Parmesan cheese or crumbled goat cheese.

MAKES 6 SERVINGS

1 medium eggplant, diced

1 medium onion, diced

1 (15-oz.) jar roasted red bell peppers, well drained and
  cut into small pieces

3 large cloves garlic, minced

2 (14 1/2-oz.) cans fat-free chicken broth

1/2 cup vermouth or dry white wine

1 cup day-old French bread cubes

1/2 teaspoon dried oregano leaves, crushed

1/2 teaspoon dried thyme leaves, crushed

1/2 teaspoon salt

1/2 teaspoon ground black pepper

1/4 cup minced fresh parsley

6 tablespoons crumbled goat cheese or shredded
  Parmesan cheese

Combine all ingredients, except parsley and cheese, in a 3 1/2-quart slow cooker. Mix well. Cover and cook on LOW 7 to 8 hours or until eggplant is very tender. Just before serving, stir in parsley. Ladle into soup bowls and garnish each serving with 1 tablespoon of the cheese.

Per serving: Cal 134 · Carb 21 gm · Prot 4 gm · Total fat 2.5 gm · Sat fat 1 gm · Cal from fat 22 · Chol 8 mg · Sodium 658 mg

GOLD 'N' GREEN SQUASH SOUP

*W*hen trimming leeks, remove and discard roots and thick tough green leaves. Sand can accumulate between the layers, so rinse leeks under running water.

MAKES 6 TO 8 SERVINGS

1 1/2 pounds banana squash

1 leek

1 green apple, peeled, cored, and chopped

1 orange, peeled, seeded, and cut into chunks

2 (14 1/2-oz.) cans fat-free chicken broth

1/4 teaspoon salt

1/8 teaspoon ground black pepper

1 teaspoon chopped fresh thyme

Several drops of hot sauce (optional)

Chopped chives

Peel squash and cut into about 1-inch pieces. Trim leek, quarter lengthwise, and wash to remove dirt. Cut leek into 1/2-inch pieces. Combine squash, leek, apple, orange, broth, salt, pepper, and thyme in a 3 1/2-quart slow cooker. Cover and cook on LOW about 6 hours or until vegetables are tender.

Puree soup mixture, in batches, in a blender or food processor. Add hot sauce, if using. Ladle into soup bowls. Sprinkle each serving with chopped chives.

Per serving: Cal 86 · Carb 21 gm · Prot 2 gm · Total fat 0 gm · Sat fat 0 gm · Cal from fat 0 · Chol 0 mg · Sodium 267 mg

FENNEL AND POTATO SOUP

*F*ennel, called *finocchio* in some Italian markets, has a sweet, mild aniselike flavor.

MAKES 5 OR 6 SERVINGS

1 fennel bulb

2 (14 1/2-oz.) cans fat-free chicken broth

3 medium potatoes, peeled and diced

1/2 cup chopped celery

1 small onion, chopped

1/2 teaspoon salt

1/8 teaspoon ground black pepper

Chop feathery fennel leaves and save for garnish. Trim fennel. Remove tough base and discard. Quarter bulb and chop into small strips. Combine fennel in a 3 1/2-quart slow cooker with chicken broth, potatoes, celery, onion, salt, and pepper. Cover and cook on LOW about 8 hours or until vegetables are tender.

Ladle into soup bowls. Sprinkle each serving with reserved fennel leaves.

Per serving: Cal 90 · Carb 19 gm · Prot 4 gm · Total fat 0 gm · Sat fat 0 gm · Cal from fat 0 · Chol 0 mg · Sodium 651 mg

GINGERED CARROT SOUP

*I*f your food processor can't handle all the vegetables at one time, divide them in half and process half at a time.

MAKES 5 OR 6 SERVINGS

8 medium carrots, peeled and cut into 1-inch chunks

1 medium potato, peeled and cut into 1-inch chunks

1 small onion, coarsely chopped

2 teaspoons grated gingerroot

2 tablespoons light brown sugar

1/2 teaspoon salt

1/8 teaspoon ground black pepper

1 (14 1/2-oz.) can fat-free chicken broth

1/4 teaspoon grated lemon peel

1 (5-oz.) can evaporated skim milk

Combine carrots, potato, onion, gingerroot, brown sugar, salt, pepper, and broth in a 3 1/2-quart slow cooker. Cover and cook on LOW about 10 hours or until vegetables are tender.

Process vegetables with a little broth in a food processor or blender until coarsely chopped; return to slow cooker. Turn control to HIGH. Stir in lemon peel and milk. Cover and heat until hot, about 30 minutes. Ladle into soup bowls.

Per serving: Cal 128 · Carb 27 gm · Prot 5 gm · Total fat 0 gm · Sat fat 0 gm · Cal from fat 0 · Chol 1 mg · Sodium 496 mg

CURRIED LENTIL-LEEK SOUP

*P*resoaking is not necessary with lentils; just combine ingredients and cook in a slow cooker.

MAKES 6 OR 7 SERVINGS

3/4 cup dried lentils

1 (28-oz.) can crushed tomatoes

1 teaspoon curry powder

2 tablespoons chopped fresh basil

1/4 teaspoon salt

1/8 teaspoon ground black pepper

1 leek, thinly sliced

2 (14 1/2-oz.) cans fat-free chicken broth

Combine all ingredients in a 3 1/2-quart slow cooker. Cover and cook on LOW 6 1/2 to 7 hours or until lentils are tender.

Ladle into soup bowls.

Per serving: Cal 85 · Carb 19 gm · Prot 7 gm · Total fat 0.5 gm · Sat fat 0 gm · Cal from fat 5 · Chol 0 mg · Sodium 662 mg

CHICKEN 'N' VEGETABLE SOUP WITH FRESH SALSA

*I*t is easy to double the recipe for a potluck supper.

MAKES 4 OR 5 SERVINGS

2 chicken thighs

2 potatoes, peeled and diced

2 ears of corn

3 cups fat-free chicken broth or bouillon

4 to 5 fresh mushrooms, sliced

1/4 teaspoon salt

Fresh Salsa

1 small tomato, diced

1 jalapeño chile, chopped

1 green onion, chopped

1/2 small avocado, peeled, pitted and chopped

Remove and discard skin and bones from chicken; finely chop. Combine chicken and potatoes in a 3 1/2-quart slow cooker. Remove husks and silk from corn. Cut off kernels and add to slow cooker. Stir in broth, mushrooms, and salt. Cover and cook on LOW about 4 hours or until potatoes are tender.

Prepare salsa: Combine all ingredients in a small bowl. Spoon soup into individual bowls. Top each serving with salsa.

Per serving: Cal 201 · Carb 28 gm · Prot 13 gm · Total fat 6 gm · Sat fat 1 gm · Cal from fat 54 · Chol 28 mg · Sodium 598 mg

TURKEY TORTILLA SOUP

*T*his substantial soup can be used as a hearty main dish for lunch or supper.

MAKES 8 SERVINGS

2 medium turkey thighs

1 (15- or 16-oz.) can diced tomatoes in juice

1 medium onion, diced

1 clove garlic, crushed

1 to 2 jalapeño chiles, seeded and chopped

2 (14 1/2-oz.) cans fat-free chicken broth

1/2 teaspoon salt

4 corn tortillas, cut into 1/4-inch strips

Chopped cilantro

Remove and discard skin and fat from turkey. Combine turkey, tomatoes, onion, garlic, jalapeño chiles, broth, and salt in a 3 1/2-quart slow cooker. Cover and cook on LOW 7 to 8 hours or until turkey is tender. Meanwhile, preheat oven to 400F (205C). Arrange tortilla strips in a single layer on a 15 x 10-inch baking sheet. Toast tortillas in oven 6 to 8 minutes or until golden, stirring once; set aside.

Remove turkey from slow cooker and cool slightly. Remove bones from turkey. Chop turkey; divide among soup bowls. Process remaining soup mixture in a blender or food processor until pureed. Pour over turkey in soup bowls. Top each serving with tortilla strips and cilantro.

Per serving: Cal 77 · Carb 10 gm · Prot 6 gm · Total fat 1 gm · Sat fat 0 gm · Cal from fat 9 · Chol 11 mg · Sodium 518 mg

1/2 C 1P

ITALIAN SAUSAGE
AND VEGETABLE CHOWDER

*C*anned tomatoes usually add a richer flavor to your soup as the tomatoes are harvested and canned at their peak.

MAKES 7 OR 8 SERVINGS

1/2 pound (3 links) hot Italian turkey sausage

1 (28-oz.) can ready-cut tomatoes

4 cups hot water

1/2 cup dry red wine

2 teaspoons instant beef bouillon granules

1 medium onion, chopped

1 large clove garlic, peeled

1 (15-oz.) can garbanzo beans with liquid

2 cups lightly packed chopped green cabbage

1/4 pound fresh green beans, cut into 1-inch pieces
    (about 1 cup)

1 medium carrot, peeled and diced

1 teaspoon dry Italian seasoning, crushed

1 teaspoon salt

1/4 teaspoon ground black pepper

1 large zucchini, cut into 1/2-inch cubes

1 cup small elbow macaroni

1/4 cup grated Parmesan cheese (optional)

1/4 cup minced fresh parsley (optional)

Remove casing from sausage links. Cut into 1-inch-thick slices; set aside. Combine tomatoes, hot water, wine, beef bouillon granules, onion, garlic, garbanzo beans, cabbage, green beans, carrot, Italian seasoning, salt, and pepper in a 4-quart slow cooker. Gently stir in sausage slices. Cover and cook on LOW 8 to 9 hours or until vegetables are almost tender.

Turn control to HIGH; add zucchini and macaroni. Stir, re-cover, and cook on HIGH 30 to 45 minutes longer or until zucchini and macaroni are tender.

Ladle into soup bowls. Sprinkle each serving with Parmesan cheese and minced parsley, if desired.

Per serving: Cal 228 · Carb 33 gm · Prot 13 gm · Total fat 5 gm · Sat fat 1 gm · Cal from fat 45 · Chol 17 mg · Sodium 1100 mg *2c 1½ P*

BLACK-EYED PEA SOUP

A green salad and a roll make this a satisfying meal.

MAKES 8 OR 9 SERVINGS

1 pound dried black-eyed peas

1/2 pound 97% fat-free smoked ham, cut into 1/2-inch
cubes (2 cups)

1 medium onion, diced

4 small carrots, peeled and sliced into 1/4-inch-thick
rounds

1 1/2 cups sliced celery

2 dried red chiles

2 small bay leaves

1 1/2 tablespoons imitation bacon bits

1/2 teaspoon dried thyme leaves, crushed

1/4 teaspoon ground black pepper

10 cups hot water

1 teaspoon salt or to taste

1/3 cup minced fresh parsley

Sort peas and rinse. Place peas in a 6-quart slow cooker. Add remaining ingredients, except salt and minced parsley. Cover and cook on LOW 10 to 12 hours or until peas are tender. Stir in salt and parsley. Ladle into soup bowls.

Per serving: Cal 248 · Carb 41 gm · Prot 19 gm · Total fat 2 gm · Sat fat 0 gm · Cal from fat 18 · Chol 18 mg · Sodium 676 mg

DOUBLE-CORN STEW

*T*his hearty stew is enhanced by the flavors of fresh corn and tomatoes.

MAKES 4 OR 5 SERVINGS

2 ears of corn

1 (14- to 15-oz.) can golden hominy, drained

1 medium onion, finely chopped

2 medium tomatoes, chopped

1 (14 1/2-oz.) can fat-free chicken broth

1/4 teaspoon ground black pepper

4 to 5 ounces ham steak or baked ham, coarsely
  chopped

Chopped cilantro

Remove husks and silk from corn. Cut off kernels and add to a slow cooker. Stir in hominy, onion, tomatoes, broth, pepper, and ham. Cover and cook on LOW 5 to 6 hours or until vegetables are tender.

Ladle into soup bowls. Sprinkle each serving with cilantro.

Per serving: Cal 156 · Carb 23 gm · Prot 11 gm · Total fat 3 gm · Sat fat 1 gm · Cal from fat 27 · Chol 15 mg · Sodium 752 mg

HEARTY CONFETTI FISH CHOWDER

*I*mitation bacon bits add a slight smoky flavor without adding extra fat.

MAKES 6 TO 8 SERVINGS

2 medium potatoes, peeled and cut into 1/4-inch cubes

2 medium carrots, peeled and thinly sliced

1 stalk celery, thinly sliced

1 small leek, trimmed and thinly sliced

2 cloves garlic, minced

3 cups water

1/2 cup dry white wine

2 tablespoons imitation bacon bits

3/4 teaspoon salt

1/4 teaspoon ground white pepper

1/4 teaspoon ground thyme

1 teaspoon Worcestershire sauce

1/4 to 1/2 teaspoon hot sauce

1/3 cup dry nonfat milk powder

1/4 cup all-purpose flour

1/2 cup water

3/4 pound firm white fish, cut into 1/2-inch cubes

1 (2-oz.) jar chopped pimientos, drained

Combine potatoes, carrots, celery, leek, garlic, water, wine, imitation bacon bits, salt, pepper, thyme, Worcestershire sauce, and hot sauce in a 3 1/2-quart slow cooker. Cover and cook on LOW 7 to 8 hours or until potatoes are tender.

Turn control to HIGH. In a small bowl, combine dry milk powder and flour. Gradually whisk in water; stir into mixture in slow cooker. Add fish and pimientos. Cover and cook on HIGH 15 to 20 minutes or until fish flakes easily with a fork and chowder is slightly thickened.

Ladle into soup bowls.

Per serving: Cal 181 · Carb 23 gm · Prot 16 gm · Total fat 1 gm · Sat fat 0 gm · Cal from fat 9 · Chol 22 mg · Sodium 432 mg

SMOKED SAUSAGE CHOWDER

*A*dd the larger amount of red pepper flakes if you like spicy chowder.

MAKES 5 OR 6 SERVINGS

1/4 pound light Polish kielbasa, chopped

1 cup mild green chile picante sauce

1 clove garlic, finely chopped

1 (10-oz.) package frozen whole-kernel corn, thawed

1 medium tomato, chopped

1 (14 1/2-oz.) can fat-free chicken broth

1 (15 1/2-oz.) can garbanzo beans, drained

1 tablespoon chopped fresh cilantro

1/8 to 1/4 teaspoon crushed dried red pepper flakes

Combine all ingredients in a 3 1/2-quart slow cooker. Cover and cook on LOW 3 to 4 hours.

Ladle into soup bowls.

Per serving: Cal 185 · Carb 33 gm · Prot 11 gm · Total fat 2 gm · Sat fat 1 gm · Cal from fat 18 · Chol 10 mg · Sodium 1100 mg

MINESTRONE STEW

Serve with thick slices of French bread for a hearty lunch or dinner.

MAKES ABOUT 8 SERVINGS

1/2 pound boneless beef chuck steak, cut into 1/2-inch cubes

1 medium onion, diced

1 (14 1/2-oz.) can beef broth

1 (28-oz.) can tomatoes, chopped

1 tablespoon chopped fresh parsley

1 tablespoon chopped fresh basil

1 (16-oz.) can garbanzo beans, drained

1/4 head cabbage, shredded (about 3 cups)

1/2 teaspoon salt

1/8 teaspoon ground black pepper

1 cup small elbow macaroni

2 tablespoons grated Romano or Parmesan cheese (optional)

Combine beef, onion, broth, tomatoes, parsley, basil, beans, cabbage, salt, and pepper in a 3 1/2-quart slow cooker. Cover and cook on LOW about 8 hours or until beef is tender. Cook macaroni according to package directions; drain and stir into contents of slow cooker. Spoon into soup bowls. Sprinkle with cheese, if desired.

Per serving: Cal 227 · Carb 25 gm · Prot 13 gm · Total fat 8 gm · Sat fat 0 gm · Cal from fat 72 · Chol 24 mg · Sodium 705 mg

BEEF AND BULGUR CHILI CALIENTE

*B*ulgur wheat adds a chewy texture that tricks the palate into thinking the chili is rich with meat.

MAKES 7 OR 8 SERVINGS

1/2 pound extra-lean ground beef

1/4 cup bulgur wheat

3 to 4 tablespoons chili powder

1 tablespoon beef bouillon granules

1 teaspoon ground cumin

1 teaspoon dried oregano leaves, crushed

1/2 teaspoon salt

1/4 teaspoon ground black pepper

3 large cloves garlic, minced

2 large stalks celery, diced

1 medium onion, diced

1/2 cup diced green bell pepper

1 to 2 tablespoons hot sauce

1 (28-oz.) can diced tomatoes with juice

1 (27-oz.) can red kidney beans, undrained

1 (7-oz.) can whole green chiles, drained and cut into
   large chunks

1/4 cup tequila (optional)

Crumble meat into a slow cooker. Add bulgur wheat. Sprinkle with chili powder, bouillon granules, cumin, oregano, salt, and black pepper; mix well. Add garlic, celery, onion, bell pepper, hot sauce, tomatoes, and beans with liquid. Mix well. Cover and cook on LOW 8 to 10 hours or until meat is tender.

Stir in chiles and tequila, if using. Cover and cook 20 to 30 minutes for flavors to blend. Ladle into individual bowls.

Per serving: Cal 244 · Carb 33 gm · Prot 15 gm · Total fat 7 gm · Sat fat 2 gm · Cal from fat 63 · Chol 22 mg · Sodium 784 mg

BLOND CHILI

*B*reak tradition with a chili featuring yellow tomatoes and trendy cannellini beans, accented with crunchy jicama.

MAKES 6 OR 7 SERVINGS

3/4 pound breakfast turkey sausage links, cut into thirds

12 dried yellow or red tomato halves, coarsely chopped

3 or 4 shallots, peeled and chopped

1 small jicama, peeled and julienned

1 (4-oz.) can chopped green chiles, drained

1/4 teaspoon ground cumin

1/4 teaspoon ground chili powder

1/4 teaspoon dried oregano

1/4 teaspoon salt

1/8 teaspoon ground black pepper

2 (15-oz.) cans cannellini beans, drained

1 (14 1/2-oz.) can fat-free chicken broth

2 ounces reduced-fat mozzarella cheese, shredded
  (1/2 cup)

Combine all ingredients except cheese in a 3 1/2-quart slow cooker. Cover and cook on LOW 4 1/2 to 5 hours or until tomatoes are tender. Ladle into individual bowls and sprinkle each serving with mozzarella cheese.

Per serving: Cal 246 · Carb 26 gm · Prot 19 gm · Total fat 8 gm · Sat fat 1 gm · Cal from fat 72 · Chol 47 mg · Sodium 665 mg

CORN 'N' BEAN CHILI

A hearty, filling main dish with less meat than traditional chilies.

MAKES 6 SERVINGS

3/4 pound lean boneless beef chuck, chopped

1 medium onion, chopped

1 clove garlic, crushed

1 red bell pepper, chopped

1 (27-oz.) can red kidney beans, drained and rinsed

1/2 teaspoon chili powder

1/4 teaspoon ground sage

1/4 teaspoon ground cinnamon

1 (11-oz.) can whole-kernel corn, undrained

1 (4-oz.) can chopped green chiles, drained

1/4 cup low-fat plain yogurt

Chopped cilantro

Crumble meat into a 3 1/2-quart slow cooker. Add onion, garlic, bell pepper, beans, chili powder, sage, cinnamon, corn with liquid, and chiles. Cover and cook on LOW 6 1/2 to 7 hours or until meat is tender.

Ladle into individual bowls. Top each serving with yogurt, then with chopped cilantro.

Per serving: Cal 250 · Carb 26 gm · Prot 15 gm · Total fat 10 gm · Sat fat 4 gm · Cal from fat 90 · Chol 22 mg · Sodium 426 mg

BLACK AND WHITE CHILI
WITH PORK

*T*his interesting two-color bean dish has a delightful flavor.

MAKES 6 SERVINGS

3/4 pound boneless pork, cut into 1/2-inch cubes

1 (15-oz.) can black beans, drained and rinsed

1 (15-oz.) can small white beans, drained and rinsed

1 red or yellow bell pepper, chopped

1 medium tomato, peeled, seeded, and chopped

1 small onion, thinly sliced

1 clove garlic, crushed

1 teaspoon ground cumin

1 tablespoon chili powder

1 (8-oz.) can tomato sauce

1/3 cup low-fat yogurt or sour cream

2 tablespoons chopped fresh cilantro

Combine pork, beans, bell pepper, tomato, onion, garlic, cumin, chili powder, and tomato sauce in a 3 1/2-quart slow cooker. Cover and cook on LOW about 6 hours or until pork is tender.

Ladle into individual bowls. Spoon about 1 tablespoon yogurt or sour cream on top of each bowl; sprinkle with cilantro.

Per serving: Cal 269 · Carb 30 gm · Prot 22 gm · Total fat 6 gm · Sat fat 2 gm · Cal from fat 54 · Chol 39 mg · Sodium 363 mg

HOMINY AND BEEF SAUSAGE CHILI

*T*his is a shortcut variation of a favorite traditional family recipe.

MAKES 8 TO 10 SERVINGS

1/2 pound smoked beef sausage, coarsely chopped

1 medium onion, chopped

1 clove garlic, crushed

1 jalapeño chile, seeded and chopped

1 (15-oz.) can yellow hominy, drained

1 (15-oz.) can white hominy, drained

1 (15-oz.) can Louisiana-style red beans, undrained

Combine all ingredients in a 3 1/2-quart slow cooker. Cover and cook on LOW about 7 hours or until onion is tender.

Ladle into individual bowls.

Per serving: Cal 136 · Carb 19 gm · Prot 10 gm · Total fat 1 gm · Sat fat 0.5 gm · Cal from fat 9 · Chol 13 mg · Sodium 609 mg

LAMB AND BLACK BEAN CHILI

*T*he well-seasoned combination of lamb and black beans makes this a chili worth trying.

MAKES 4 TO 6 SERVINGS

3/4 pound boneless lean lamb, cut into 1-inch cubes

1 clove garlic, finely chopped

1 medium onion, chopped

1 tablespoon chili powder

2 teaspoons chopped fresh oregano leaves

1/4 teaspoon salt

1 tablespoon chopped fresh cilantro

2 (15-oz.) cans black beans, drained

2 (14 1/2-oz.) cans stewed tomatoes with bell pepper and onion, undrained

Combine lamb, garlic, onion, chili powder, oregano, salt, and cilantro in a 3 1/2-quart slow cooker. Stir in beans and tomatoes. Cover and cook on LOW about 7 hours or until lamb is tender.

Ladle into individual bowls.

Per serving: Cal 234 · Carb 25 gm · Prot 24 gm · Total fat 4 gm · Sat fat 1 gm · Cal from fat 36 · Chol 54 mg · Sodium 902 mg

TURKEY SAUSAGE CHILI
WITH BEANS

*T*urkey sausage provides an exciting flavor that is slightly different from that of traditional chili, as well as a lower fat content.

MAKES 6 SERVINGS

14 to 16 ounces turkey breakfast sausage, diced

1 (28-oz.) can cut tomatoes in juice

1 jalapeño chile, seeded and finely chopped

1 onion, chopped

1 clove garlic, crushed

2 teaspoons chili powder

1 teaspoon low-sodium beef bouillon granules

1 (27-oz.) can red kidney beans, drained

2 tablespoons low-fat yogurt

2 tablespoons chopped fresh cilantro

Thoroughly combine turkey sausage, tomatoes, jalapeño chile, onion, garlic, chili powder, and beef bouillon granules in a 3 1/2-quart slow cooker. Stir in beans. Cover and cook on LOW about 6 hours or until onion is tender.

Ladle into individual bowls. Top each serving with about 1 teaspoon of yogurt, then chopped cilantro.

Per serving: Cal 265 · Carb 33 gm · Prot 20 gm · Total fat 8 gm · Sat fat 0 gm · Cal from fat 72 · Chol 49 mg · Sodium 920 mg

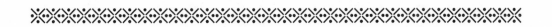

AROUND THE WORLD WITH CHICKEN

*I*n many countries around the world, chicken is one of the most popular main dishes. Here at home, it has been one of our staples for entertaining as well as for family meals. The slow cooker makes it even more popular. Working mothers like the idea of nourishing and satisfying food that's ready when the family returns home from school or work.

Favorites range from traditional chicken that's stuffed with mashed potatoes and celery to one with a slight Asian accent that's filled with a water-chestnut mixture and brushed with soy sauce. For those with fond memories of grandma's kitchen, there's a traditional Old-Fashioned Chicken 'n' Noodles.

Cooking Tip

An easy way to test poultry for doneness is to use an instant-read thermometer. Ground chicken or turkey should be cooked to an internal temperature of 165F (75C) and a whole chicken or turkey, or chicken or turkey part, should be cooked to 180F (80C). Stuffing should be cooked to 165F (75C).

ROASTED CHICKEN WITH ROSEMARY AND GARLIC

*F*resh rosemary and garlic add great flavor to the chicken.

MAKES ABOUT 6 SERVINGS

1 (4-to 5-lb.) whole roasting chicken

8 small sprigs of fresh rosemary

4 cloves garlic, halved

Remove excess fat from chicken. Remove giblets from chicken and refrigerate for another use. Rinse and drain chicken. Starting at neck cavity, carefully loosen skin from breast with your fingers or a knife by gently pushing between the skin and meat. Insert 2 garlic pieces and 2 rosemary sprigs under breast skin at edge of wings. Continue pulling skin and insert 2 rosemary sprigs and 2 garlic pieces under drumstick skin. Make a small slit in skin on each wing. Insert a garlic piece and a rosemary sprig into each. Insert 2 garlic pieces and 2 rosemary sprigs in body cavity. Tie legs together and wings close to body.

Place chicken, breast side down, in a 4- or 5-quart slow cooker. Cover and cook on LOW 6 or 7 hours or until juices are clear when thick part of chicken is pierced with a knife.

Remove chicken from slow cooker and discard garlic and rosemary. Cut chicken into individual pieces and serve.

Per serving: Cal 198 · Carb 1 gm · Prot 26 gm · Total fat 9 gm · Sat fat 3 gm · Cal from fat 81 · Chol 55 mg · Sodium 92 mg

POTATO- AND CELERY-STUFFED CHICKEN

*T*his was a traditional family favorite at my friend Grace Wheeler's house when her children were growing up.

MAKES 4 TO 6 SERVINGS

1 (2 1/2- to 3-lb.) whole broiler-fryer chicken

1 cup instant mashed-potato flakes

1 cup finely chopped celery

1/4 cup finely chopped onion

1 tablespoon minced fresh parsley

2 tablespoons margarine, melted

1/2 teaspoon poultry seasoning

1/4 teaspoon salt

1/4 teaspoon ground black pepper

2 teaspoons olive oil

1 clove garlic, minced

Paprika, salt, and ground black pepper for seasoning

1 tablespoon cornstarch

Remove excess fat from chicken. Remove giblets from chicken and refrigerate for another use. Rinse and drain chicken. In a small bowl, combine potato flakes, celery, onion, parsley, margarine, poultry seasoning, salt, and pepper. Spoon into chicken cavities. Secure openings with wooden picks. Tie legs together and wings close to body. Combine olive oil and garlic; rub on outside of chicken. Sprinkle with paprika, salt, and pepper.

Place chicken, breast side up, in slow cooker. Cover and cook on LOW 5 to 6 hours or until juices are clear when thick part of chicken is pierced with a knife.

Remove chicken from cooker. Pour drippings into a 2-cup glass measuring cup; add enough water to equal 1 cup. Stir in cornstarch. Microwave on HIGH, stirring once, about 1 1/2 minutes, or until slightly thickened. Skim off excess fat. Remove string and wooden picks from chicken. Carve and serve with dressing and gravy.

Per serving: Cal 589 · Carb 18 gm · Prot 58 gm · Total fat 30 gm · Sat fat 7 gm · Cal from fat 270 · Chol 124 mg · Sodium 456 mg

ROASTED CHICKEN STUFFED WITH WATER CHESTNUTS AND BEAN SPROUTS

*I*f roasting chickens are not available at your market, purchase a large whole fryer.

MAKES 4 TO 6 SERVINGS

1 (5-lb.) whole roasting chicken

3 tablespoons soy sauce

1 (8-oz.) can water chestnuts, drained and chopped

1 cup (about 3 oz.) fresh bean sprouts

1/2 cup chopped celery

1 slice bread, toasted and chopped

Remove excess fat from chicken. Remove giblets from chicken and refrigerate for another use. Rinse and drain chicken. Set aside 1 tablespoon of the soy sauce. Combine remaining 2 tablespoons soy sauce with water chestnuts, bean sprouts, celery, and bread. Stuff mixture into chicken.

Place chicken, breast side down, in a 4- or 5-quart slow cooker. Brush chicken with reserved 1 tablespoon soy sauce. Cover and cook on LOW 4 or 5 hours or until juices are clear when thick part of chicken is pierced with a knife. Carve chicken and serve with stuffing.

Per serving: Cal 363 · Carb 9 gm · Prot 51 gm · Total fat 12 gm · Sat fat 3 gm · Cal from fat 108 · Chol 94 mg · Sodium 711 mg ½c 7P

HONEY-HOISIN CHICKEN

*T*he combination of Oriental ingredients with traditional seasonings results in an exciting flavor for an attractive main dish.

MAKES 5 OR 6 SERVINGS

2 1/2 to 3 pounds chicken pieces

2 tablespoons soy sauce

2 tablespoons hoisin sauce

2 tablespoons honey

2 tablespoons dry white wine

1 tablespoon grated gingerroot

1/4 teaspoon salt

1/8 teaspoon ground black pepper

2 tablespoons cornstarch

2 tablespoons cold water

Sesame seeds, toasted (see Note, page 55)

Rinse chicken and pat dry with paper towels. Combine soy sauce, hoisin sauce, honey, wine, ginger, salt, and pepper. Dip each piece of chicken into sauce; then place in a 3 1/2-quart slow cooker. Pour remaining sauce over chicken. Cover and cook on LOW about 4 or 5 hours or until chicken is tender.

Turn control to HIGH. Remove chicken from slow cooker and keep warm. Dissolve cornstarch in cold water. Stir mixture into juices in slow cooker. Cover and cook on HIGH 15 to 20 minutes or until slightly thickened. Spoon sauce over chicken and sprinkle with sesame seeds.

Per serving: Cal 243 · Carb 11 gm · Prot 30 gm · Total fat 7 gm · Sat fat 2 gm · Cal from fat 63 · Chol 56 mg · Sodium 630 mg *1/2 c 4P*

CHICKEN AND MANGO WITH GINGER-CURRY TOPPING

A combination of popular tropical flavors results in a new way to present chicken.

MAKES 5 OR 6 SERVINGS

1 large mango

2 teaspoons fresh lemon juice

1 teaspoon honey

1 clove garlic, crushed

1/8 teaspoon paprika

1/4 teaspoon salt

1/8 teaspoon ground black pepper

2 1/2 to 3 pounds chicken pieces

Ginger-Curry Topping

1/3 cup plain low-fat yogurt

1/4 teaspoon curry powder

1/4 teaspoon grated gingerroot

1 teaspoon brown sugar

1/8 teaspoon grated orange peel

Peel mango and remove flesh from seed; mash in a small bowl. Stir in lemon juice, honey, garlic, paprika, salt, and pepper. Rinse chicken and pat dry with paper towels. Place chicken in a 3 1/2-quart slow cooker. Spoon mango mixture over chicken. Cover and cook on LOW about 4 hours or until chicken is tender.

While chicken cooks, make topping: Combine yogurt, curry powder, gingerroot, brown sugar, and orange peel in a small bowl; refrigerate.

To serve, arrange chicken in a serving dish and spoon drippings over chicken. Top each serving with a dab of Ginger Curry Topping.

Per serving: Cal 333 · Carb 9 gm · Prot 38 gm · Total fat 15 gm · Sat fat 4 gm · Cal from fat 135 · Chol 83 mg · Sodium 236 mg

OLD-FASHIONED CHICKEN 'N' NOODLES

*R*eminiscent of grandma's house, this dish is easy to put together in your slow cooker.

MAKES 6 TO 8 SERVINGS

2 1/2 to 3 pounds chicken pieces

1 small onion, finely chopped

1/2 cup thinly sliced celery

1 clove garlic, minced

1/2 teaspoon salt

1/8 teaspoon ground black pepper

1/2 teaspoon poultry seasoning

1/2 teaspoon chopped fresh thyme

1 (10 1/2-oz.) can condensed chicken broth

1/4 cup cornstarch

1/3 cup cold water

8 to 12 ounces medium egg noodles

Chopped fresh parsley

Rinse chicken and pat dry with paper towels. Combine chicken, onion, celery, garlic, salt, pepper, poultry seasoning, and thyme in a 3 1/2-quart slow cooker. Add chicken broth. Cover and cook on low 4 or 5 hours or until chicken is tender.

Remove chicken from slow cooker. Discard skin and bones; cut chicken into bite-size pieces and set aside.

Turn control to HIGH. Dissolve cornstarch in cold water. Stir into juices in slow cooker. Cover and cook on HIGH 15 to 20 minutes or until slightly thickened. Stir in chicken.

Meanwhile, cook noodles according to package directions and drain. Spoon mixture over cooked noodles. Sprinkle with chopped parsley.

Per serving: Cal 477 · Carb 35 gm · Prot 45 gm · Total fat 16 gm · Sat fat 4 gm · Cal from fat 144 · Chol 83 mg · Sodium 638 mg

PLUM-GLAZED CHICKEN

*T*ender pieces of chicken are seasoned with a sweet-sour plum sauce.

MAKES 5 OR 6 SERVINGS

2 1/2 to 3 pounds chicken pieces, skinned

1/2 cup plum preserves

1/4 cup minced onion

1 clove garlic, minced

3 tablespoons chili sauce

2 tablespoons balsamic vinegar

1 tablespoon soy sauce

1/2 teaspoon ground ginger

1/4 teaspoon ground allspice

1/4 teaspoon ground black pepper

1 tablespoon cornstarch

2 tablespoons dry sherry

Hot cooked rice

Diagonally sliced green onions, including some tops

Rinse chicken and pat dry with paper towels. Place half of chicken in a 3 1/2-quart slow cooker. In a small bowl, combine preserves, onion, garlic, chili sauce, vinegar, soy sauce, ginger, allspice, and pepper. Spoon half of the mixture over chicken in slow cooker. Top with remaining chicken; then remaining preserves mixture. Cover and cook on LOW 7 to 8 hours or until chicken is tender.

Arrange chicken pieces over hot cooked rice. Skim fat from cooking juices and discard. Pour remaining liquid into a small saucepan. Dissolve cornstarch in sherry. Stir into cooking juices; cook, stirring constantly, over medium-high heat until thickened slightly. Pour glaze over chicken and sprinkle with green onions.

Per serving: Cal 478 · Carb 29 gm · Prot 46 gm · Total fat 17 gm · Sat fat 5 gm · Cal from fat 153 · Chol 99 mg · Sodium 496 mg

ORANGE AND GINGER CHICKEN

*T*he flavors of this dish are similar to those of favorite traditional Oriental chicken recipes but require a lot less work.

MAKES 5 OR 6 SERVINGS

2 to 3 pounds chicken pieces

1 (8-oz.) can sliced water chestnuts, drained

1/2 cup orange juice

1 teaspoon grated orange peel

3 tablespoons soy sauce

2 teaspoons grated gingerroot

1 clove garlic, crushed

3 tablespoons cornstarch

3 tablespoons cold water

Cooked rice

Rinse chicken and pat dry with paper towels. Place chicken pieces in a 3 1/2-quart slow cooker. Top with water chestnuts. In a small bowl, combine orange juice, orange peel, soy sauce, ginger, and garlic. Pour over chicken. Cover and cook on low about 4 hours or until chicken is tender.

Remove chicken and water chestnuts and keep warm. Dissolve cornstarch in water; stir into cooking juices in slow cooker. Cover and cook on HIGH, stirring occasionally, 10 to 15 minutes or until slightly thickened. Spoon sauce over chicken and rice.

Per serving without rice: Cal 362 · Carb 14 gm · Prot 36 gm · Total fat 17 gm · Sat fat 5 gm · Cal from fat 153 · Chol 83 mg · Sodium 758 mg

✳ CHICKEN WITH CABBAGE AND APPLES

$\mathcal{R}$ice or noodles are the perfect accompaniment for dishes with oriental-accented seasonings.

MAKES ABOUT 5 SERVINGS

3 to 3 1/2 pounds chicken pieces

1/2 head cabbage, shredded (about 3 cups)

1 small onion, sliced

2 apples, cored and cut into wedges

2 tablespoons soy sauce

2 teaspoons grated fresh gingerroot

1/8 teaspoon red pepper flakes

Rinse chicken and pat dry with paper towels. Place cabbage in bottom of a 3 1/2-quart slow cooker. Top with onion, chicken, and apples. Combine soy sauce, ginger, and pepper flakes. Spoon over chicken and vegetables. Cover and cook on LOW about 6 hours or until chicken is tender.

Per serving: Cal 492 · Carb 13 gm · Prot 55 gm · Total fat 23 gm · Sat fat 6 gm · Cal from fat 207 · Chol 122 mg · Sodium 622 mg

CRANBERRY-ORANGE CHICKEN

To reduce fat, remove and discard the skin from the chicken before cooking.

MAKES ABOUT 6 SERVINGS

2 1/2 to 3 pounds chicken pieces

1 (8-oz.) can whole-berry cranberry sauce

2 tablespoons orange juice

1 teaspoon grated orange peel

1/8 teaspoon ground nutmeg

1 tablespoon sweet-hot mustard

1/2 teaspoon salt

1/8 teaspoon ground black pepper

3 tablespoons cornstarch

3 tablespoons cold water

Rinse chicken and pat dry with paper towels. Place cut-up chicken in a 3 1/2-quart slow cooker. In small bowl, combine cranberry sauce, orange juice and peel, nutmeg, mustard, salt, and pepper. Stir until blended but not smooth. Pour over chicken. Cover and cook on LOW for 4 or 5 hours or until chicken is tender.

Remove chicken and keep warm. Turn control to HIGH. Dissolve cornstarch in water. Stir into pot with juices. Cook on HIGH, stirring occasionally, 10 to 15 minutes or until thickened. Spoon over chicken.

Per serving: Cal 370 · Carb 19 gm · Prot 38 gm · Total fat 14 gm · Sat fat 4 gm · Cal from fat 126 · Chol 83 mg · Sodium 333 mg

PEANUT BUTTER 'N' GINGER CHICKEN

A whisk is the best tool to efficiently mix the sauce.

MAKES 5 OR 6 SERVINGS

3 1/2 pounds chicken pieces

1/4 cup peanut butter

2 tablespoons soy sauce

1 teaspoon grated gingerroot

1/2 teaspoon grated orange peel

2 tablespoons orange juice

1/8 teaspoon hot sauce

2 green onions, including some green tops, sliced

Cooked noodles or rice

Rinse chicken and pat dry with paper towels. Place chicken in a 3 1/2-quart slow cooker. In a small bowl, whisk together peanut butter, soy sauce, ginger, orange peel, juice, and hot sauce until well blended. Stir in green onions. Spoon over chicken. Cover and cook on LOW about 5 hours or until chicken is tender.

Serve chicken over cooked noodles or rice.

Per serving without noodles: Cal 606 · Carb 4 gm · Prot 65 gm · Total fat 35 gm · Sat fat 9 gm · Cal from fat 315 · Chol 144 mg · Sodium 709 mg

CHILE-CITRUS CHICKEN WITH SUN-DRIED TOMATOES

*H*ot chile adds a spark to a traditional chicken dish that's good with noodles or rice.

MAKES 5 OR 6 SERVINGS

3 pounds chicken pieces

6 dried tomato halves, coarsely chopped

1 small dried red chile, seeded and finely chopped

2 green onions, including some tops, sliced

1/2 teaspoon salt

1/2 cup orange juice

1 teaspoon grated orange peel

2 tablespoons cornstarch

2 tablespoons cold water

Rinse chicken and pat dry with paper towels. Place chicken in a 3 1/2-quart slow cooker. In a medium bowl, combine tomatoes, chile, green onions, salt, orange juice, and orange peel. Stir until blended. Pour over chicken. Cover and cook on LOW 4 to 5 hours or until chicken is tender.

Remove chicken and keep warm. Dissolve cornstarch in water. Stir into the cooking juices in slow cooker. Cook on HIGH 15 to 20 minutes or until slightly thickened. Spoon over chicken.

Per serving: Cal 478 · Carb 9 gm · Prot 54 gm · Total fat 23 gm · Sat fat 6 gm · Cal from fat 207 · Chol 121 mg · Sodium 421 mg

PEANUTTY CHICKEN 'N' RICE

*T*he peanut mixture will be rather thick when spread on the chicken, but it is thinned down during the cooking process and can be spooned over the finished dish.

MAKES 4 TO 6 SERVINGS

3 1/2 pounds chicken pieces

1/2 cup roasted shelled peanuts

2 tablespoons soy sauce

1 clove garlic

1/8 teaspoon red pepper flakes

1 tablespoon red wine vinegar

Cooked rice

Rinse chicken and pat dry with paper towels. Place chicken in a 3 1/2-quart slow cooker. Combine peanuts, soy sauce, garlic, red pepper flakes, and red wine vinegar in a blender. Process until finely chopped. Spread sauce over chicken. Cover and cook on low about 5 hours or until chicken is tender.

Spoon chicken and cooking juices over cooked rice.

Per serving without rice: Cal 765 · Carb 5 gm · Prot 82 gm · Total fat 44 gm · Sat fat 11 gm · Cal from fat 396 · Chol 180 mg · Sodium 811 mg

RASPBERRIED DRUMSTICKS

*T*his is an ideal dish to prepare at home and take to a potluck supper.

MAKES 5 MAIN-DISH SERVINGS OR 10 POTLUCK SERVINGS

5 drumsticks with thighs attached

3 tablespoons soy sauce

1/3 cup red raspberry fruit spread or jam

1 teaspoon prepared mustard

1/4 teaspoon ground black pepper

2 tablespoons cornstarch

2 tablespoons cold water

Cooked rice

Rinse chicken and pat dry with paper towels. In a small bowl, combine soy sauce, fruit spread, mustard, and pepper. Brush soy mixture on chicken. Place chicken in a 3 1/2-quart slow cooker. Pour remaining soy mixture over chicken. Cover and cook on LOW 5 to 6 hours or until chicken is tender.

Remove chicken from slow cooker and keep warm. Turn control to HIGH. In a small bowl, dissolve cornstarch in cold water. Stir into cooking juices in slow cooker. Cook on HIGH, stirring occasionally, 10 to 15 minutes or until thickened. Spoon over chicken. Serve over cooked rice.

Per serving without rice: Cal 356 · Carb 10 gm · Prot 30 gm · Total fat 20 gm · Sat fat 6 gm · Cal from fat 180 · Chol 83 mg · Sodium 780 mg

TOUCH-OF-THE-ORIENT CHICKEN

*S*o quick and easy to put together, it cooks without any attention and is then enjoyed at dinnertime.

MAKES 5 OR 6 SERVINGS

5 or 6 chicken drumsticks with thighs attached

1/2 cup soy sauce

1/4 cup packed light brown sugar

1 clove garlic, crushed

1 (8-oz.) can tomato sauce

1 tablespoon sesame seeds, toasted (see Note below)

Rinse chicken and pat dry with paper towels. Place chicken in a 3 1/2-quart slow cooker. In a medium bowl, combine soy sauce, brown sugar, garlic, and tomato sauce. Pour sauce over chicken. Cover and cook on LOW about 5 hours or until chicken is tender.

Remove to a platter; sprinkle with sesame seeds.

Per serving: Cal 393 · Carb 17 gm · Prot 32 gm · Total fat 21 gm · Sat fat 6 gm · Cal from fat 189 · Chol 83 mg · Sodium 2055 mg

NOTE: Preheat oven to 350F (175C). Spread sesame seeds in a 9-inch pie or cake pan. Toast about 5 minutes or until golden. Or toast seeds in a dry skillet over low heat 3 or 4 minutes.

SPICED CHICKEN WITH BROWN RICE

A yogurt-orange sauce laced with an intriguing blend of spices is spooned over chicken and brown rice, giving this dish the flavors of India.

MAKES 4 OR 5 SERVINGS

6 boneless, skinless chicken thighs

1/4 teaspoon salt

1/2 teaspoon ground black pepper

1/4 teaspoon paprika

1 small onion, chopped

1 large clove garlic, finely minced or crushed

1 teaspoon sugar

1/2 teaspoon ground coriander

1/2 teaspoon ground cumin

1/8 teaspoon ground cardamom

1 1/2 teaspoons grated orange peel

1/3 cup orange juice

1 tablespoon cornstarch

1/2 cup plain nonfat yogurt

2 cups cooked brown rice

Chopped fresh cilantro

Rinse chicken and pat dry with paper towels. Remove any excess fat from chicken. Tuck ends under on each thigh to make a small bundle. Place, seam side down, on bottom of a slow cooker. Sprinkle with salt, pepper, and paprika. Combine onion, garlic, sugar, coriander, cumin, cardamom, orange peel, and orange juice in a small bowl. Spoon evenly over chicken. Cover and cook on LOW about 4 hours or until chicken is tender.

Remove chicken from slow cooker and keep warm. Pour cooking juices into a small saucepan. Combine cornstarch with yogurt in a small bowl. Stir into pan juices. Cook over medium heat, stirring constantly, until mixture thickens slightly.

Place chicken on cooked rice; spoon sauce over all. Sprinkle with cilantro.

Per serving: Cal 276 · Carb 31 gm · Prot 25 gm · Total fat 5 gm · Sat fat 1 gm · Cal from fat 45 · Chol 87 mg · Sodium 412 mg

CHICKEN WITH FRESH HERBS

*T*he chicken is seasoned with fresh herbs and layered with fresh vegetables.

MAKES 6 SERVINGS

2 leeks, sliced and rinsed

6 boneless, skinless chicken breast halves or thighs

4 ears of corn

1 large carrot, shredded

2 tomatoes, coarsely chopped

2 teaspoons chopped fresh oregano

1 teaspoon chopped fresh thyme

1/2 teaspoon salt

1/4 teaspoon ground black pepper

1 clove garlic, crushed

Place leeks on bottom of a slow cooker. Top with chicken. Cut corn kernels off the cobs. Sprinkle corn over chicken. Layer carrot over corn and chicken. Combine tomatoes, oregano, thyme, salt, pepper, and garlic in a small bowl. Spoon into slow cooker. Cover and cook on LOW about 5 hours or until chicken is tender.

Per serving: Cal 197 · Carb 15 gm · Prot 29 gm · Total fat 2 gm · Sat fat 0 gm · Cal from fat 18 · Chol 41 mg · Sodium 274 mg

CREAMY CHICKEN 'N' LEEKS

*I*f desired, use (thighs) for guests who prefer dark pieces of chicken.

MAKES 8 SERVINGS

- 8 boneless, skinless chicken breast halves
- 1/2 teaspoon salt
- 1/8 teaspoon ground black pepper
- 3 leeks, cut into 1-inch crosswise pieces and rinsed
- 1/4 cup dried currants *(or raisins)*
- 1/4 cup dry white wine
- 1/2 cup fat-free chicken broth
- 1/4 cup cornstarch
- 1/2 cup nonfat milk

Rinse chicken and pat dry with paper towels. Sprinkle chicken with salt and pepper. Place leeks in bottom of a slow cooker. Top with chicken breasts and currants. Add wine and broth. Cover and cook on LOW 6 to 7 hours or until chicken is tender.

Turn control to HIGH. Remove chicken, leeks, and currants; keep warm. In a small bowl, dissolve cornstarch in milk; gradually stir into cooking juices in slow cooker. Cover and cook on HIGH, stirring occasionally, about 15 minutes or until thickened. Serve over cooked chicken mixture.

Per serving: Cal 198 · Carb 14 gm · Prot 29 gm · Total fat 1 gm · Sat fat 0 gm · Cal from fat 9 · Chol 41 mg · Sodium 262 mg   *1C 4P*

SAVORY CHICKEN AND VEGETABLES

A delicious way to eat and enjoy your vegetables.

MAKES 5 OR 6 SERVINGS

1 pound boneless, skinless chicken breasts,
   cut into bite-size pieces

1 (16-oz.) package frozen mixed vegetables

1 small onion, chopped

1 cup sliced fresh mushrooms

1 large potato, peeled and cut into 1/4-inch cubes

1 1/4 cups water

2 tablespoons quick-cooking tapioca

1 tablespoon fresh lemon juice

2 teaspoons chicken bouillon granules

1/2 teaspoon ground white pepper

1/4 teaspoon ground mustard

1/4 teaspoon crushed sage

1/4 teaspoon salt

1/8 teaspoon garlic powder

Pinch of turmeric

1/3 cup nonfat dry milk powder

Fresh minced parsley

Rinse chicken and pat dry with paper towels. Combine chicken, mixed vegetables, onion, mushrooms, and potato in a 3 1/2-quart slow cooker. In a small bowl, combine water, tapioca, lemon juice, bouillon granules, white pepper, mustard, sage, salt, garlic powder, and turmeric. Pour over chicken mixture. Mix well. Cover and cook on LOW 6 to 7 hours.

Stir in dry milk and cook 15 minutes. Sprinkle each serving with parsley.

Per serving: Cal 237 · Carb 30 gm · Prot 26 gm · Total fat 1 gm ·
Sat fat 0 gm · Cal from fat 9 · Chol 32 mg · Sodium 225 mg

CHICKEN-VEGETABLE PINWHEELS

*B*e careful not to tear chicken with mallet when pounding it.

MAKES 6 SERVINGS

6 boneless, skinless chicken breast halves

1 egg, beaten slightly

1/4 pound Italian turkey sausage

2 slices finely chopped bread, crusts removed

1 small carrot, peeled and shredded

2 green onions, including tops, chopped

1 stalk celery, finely chopped

1/4 teaspoon salt

1/8 teaspoon fresh ground pepper

1/4 cup sliced green onions, including some tops

Rinse chicken and pat dry with paper towels. Place each breast half between waxed paper or plastic wrap. Carefully flatten chicken with meat mallet to about 1/4-inch thickness.

In a small bowl, combine egg, sausage, bread, carrot, chopped onions, celery, salt, and pepper. Spread about 1/4 cup stuffing mixture down the center of each chicken piece. Roll up; secure with a wooden pick or small skewer. Place chicken rolls in a 3 1/2-quart slow cooker. Cover and cook on LOW 4 1/2 to 5 hours. To serve, transfer chicken to plates; spoon a small amount of cooking juice over each chicken pinwheel. Garnish with green onions.

Per serving: Cal 203 · Carb 6 gm · Prot 32 gm · Total fat 4 gm · Sat fat 1 gm · Cal from fat 36 · Chol 86 mg · Sodium 377 mg

POLENTA-CHILI CASSEROLE

*I*t's easy to make your own polenta lining for a chili casserole in the slow cooker.

MAKES ABOUT 6 SERVINGS

3/4 cup yellow cornmeal

2 3/4 cups cold water

1 (15-oz.) can low-fat turkey chili with beans

1/4 cup chopped leeks

2 boneless, skinless chicken breast halves, cubed

About 1 cup (4 oz.) shredded Monterey Jack cheese

In a 2-quart saucepan, combine cornmeal and cold water. Bring to a boil over medium heat, reduce heat to low, and cook, stirring, about 5 minutes or until thickened. Remove from heat; cool about 10 minutes. Spread over bottom and 1 1/2 to 2 inches up sides of a 3 1/2-quart slow cooker.

In a medium bowl, combine turkey chili, leeks, and chicken. Spoon into center of polenta mixture. Cover and cook on LOW about 5 hours. About 15 minutes before serving, sprinkle top of bean mixture with cheese.

Per serving: Cal 255 · Carb 22 gm · Prot 19 gm · Total fat 11 gm · Sat fat 5 gm · Cal from fat 99 · Chol 42 mg · Sodium 504 mg

TUSCAN-STYLE CORNISH HENS

*T*hese are enhanced by flavorful herbs and seasonings.

MAKES 6 SERVINGS

3 Cornish hens, thawed if frozen and cut in half

2 to 3 ounces thinly sliced prosciutto, chopped

2 cloves garlic, crushed

12 fresh sage leaves, chopped

2 tablespoons chopped fresh fennel leaves

1/2 teaspoon salt

1/4 teaspoon ground pepper

2 tablespoons vegetable oil

5 teaspoons cornstarch

2 tablespoons cold water

Fresh fennel tops

Rinse hens and pat dry. In a food processor, combine prosciutto, garlic, sage, fennel, salt, pepper, and oil; process until finely chopped. Brush or pat mixture on skin and inside hens. Place hens on a trivet in a 4- to 5-quart slow cooker. Cover and cook on LOW 5 to 5 1/2 hours or until hens are tender.

Pour 1 1/2 cups cooking juices into a 2-cup measuring cup. Skim off and discard fat. In a small saucepan, dissolve cornstarch in cold water. Add cooking juices. Cook, stirring, over medium heat until slightly thickened. Spoon sauce over hens and garnish with fennel tops.

Per serving: Cal 167 · Carb 3 gm · Prot 26 gm · Total fat 5 gm · Sat fat 1 gm · Cal from fat 45 · Chol 115 mg · Sodium 383 mg

CORNISH HENS WITH FRESH SALSA

*C*ornish hens are perfect for cooking in a slow cooker. They come out moist and succulent.

MAKES 6 SERVINGS

3 Cornish hens, thawed if frozen and cut in half

1/2 teaspoon salt

1/4 teaspoon ground pepper

1/4 teaspoon seasoned salt

3 cloves garlic, cut in half

Fresh Salsa

3 medium tomatoes, peeled, seeded, and chopped

3 green onions, including tops, chopped

1/4 cup coarsely chopped fresh cilantro

2 tablespoons chopped fresh parsley

1 small jalapeño chile, seeded and finely chopped

1/4 teaspoon salt

Rinse hens and pat dry with paper towels. Season hens with salt, pepper, and seasoned salt. Insert a piece of garlic in cavity of each hen. Place hens in a 4- to 5-quart slow cooker. Cover and cook on LOW 5 to 5 1/2 hours or until hens are tender.

Meanwhile, prepare salsa: Combine all ingredients in a small bowl and refrigerate several hours for flavors to blend. Serve salsa with hens.

Per serving: Cal 157 · Carb 4 gm · Prot 24 gm · Total fat 4 gm · Sat fat 1 gm · Cal from fat 36 · Chol 110 mg · Sodium 440 mg

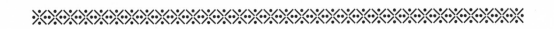

SLOW-COOKING
TURKEY DISCOVERIES

*D*uring the past few years, turkey parts have become very popular in our supermarkets. They are handy for small families or for those who don't want to worry about what to do with the remains of a huge Thanksgiving turkey.

Remember to buy turkey parts that will fit into your slow cooker. If the turkey bones make the cut too large, buy boneless parts or have the bones removed.

We have included ideas for turkey breast or cutlets and thighs as well as for plain unseasoned ground turkey and turkey sausage. Be sure to read the label on the package to determine whether additional seasonings have been added (such as in the turkey sausage).

Cooking Tip

See Cooking Tip, page 35, for tips on cooking turkey.

TURKEY WITH
JICAMA-GINGER SALSA

$\mathcal{A}$ whole turkey breast will not fit into most slow cookers, so use half of the breast or about 2 1/2 pounds.

MAKES ABOUT 6 SERVINGS

1 (2 1/2-lb.) turkey breast half with bone and skin

1/2 teaspoon salt

1/8 teaspoon ground black pepper

2 tablespoons white wine

2 stalks celery, sliced

1/4 cup chopped fresh parsley

Jicama-Ginger Salsa

1/2 cup finely chopped jicama

2 tablespoons finely chopped fresh cilantro

1/4 cup finely chopped green onions, including some tops

2 teaspoons finely chopped gingerroot

2 teaspoons finely chopped jalapeño chile

1 small tomato, peeled and finely chopped

Rinse turkey and pat dry with paper towels. Sprinkle turkey with salt and pepper. Insert meat thermometer into turkey and place in a slow cooker. Add wine. Sprinkle with celery and parsley. Cover and cook on LOW 4 to 5 hours or until turkey is tender and an instant-read thermometer registers 180F (80C).

While turkey cooks, make salsa: Combine jicama, cilantro, onions, gingerroot, jalapeño chile, and tomato in a medium bowl. Refrigerate until ready to serve.

Slice turkey and serve with salsa.

Per serving: Cal 311 · Carb 2 gm · Prot 42 gm · Total fat 13 gm · Sat fat 4 gm · Cal from fat 117 · Chol 122 mg · Sodium 308 mg

✳ TIJUANA TURKEY

*I*nspired by the flavors of mole, a popular Mexican sauce, the cocoa in this dish imparts a richness and mysterious nuance. Peanut butter replaces the usual ground nuts.

MAKES ABOUT 4 SERVINGS

1 pound turkey breast, cut into 3/4-inch cubes

1 small green bell pepper, finely chopped

1 small onion, minced

1 clove garlic, minced

1 tablespoon brown sugar

1 tablespoon chili powder

2 tablespoons cornmeal

3 tablespoons unsweetened cocoa powder

1 teaspoon ground cumin

1 teaspoon dried oregano leaves, crushed

1/2 teaspoon salt

1/4 teaspoon ground cinnamon

1/8 teaspoon ground red pepper

1 (8-oz.) can tomato sauce

1 1/2 cups water

1 1/2 tablespoons smooth peanut butter

3 cups hot cooked rice

1/4 cup chopped fresh cilantro

Combine turkey, bell pepper, onion, and garlic in a 3 1/2-quart slow cooker. In a small bowl, mix brown sugar, chili powder, cornmeal, cocoa powder, cumin, oregano, salt, cinnamon, and red pepper. Stir into turkey mixture. Whisk tomato sauce with

water and peanut butter; pour over turkey mixture, mixing well.
Cover and cook on LOW 4 to 5 hours.

Serve over hot cooked rice. Sprinkle with cilantro.

Per serving: Cal 339 · Carb 58 gm · Prot 42 gm · Total fat 5 gm ·
Sat fat 1 gm · Cal from fat 45 · Chol 90 mg · Sodium 758 mg 4C 5½P

SPINACH AND PROSCIUTTO TURKEY ROULADES

*F*or an impressive presentation, serve individual servings of sliced turkey roulade over cooked white or wild rice. (*See photo on cover.*)

MAKES 6 OR 7 SERVINGS

6 or 7 turkey cutlets (about 1 lb.)

1 (10-oz.) package chopped frozen spinach, thawed

2 tablespoons minced fresh parsley

1/4 cup dry bread crumbs

3 tablespoons shredded Parmesan cheese

3 tablespoons pine nuts, toasted (see Note, page 165)

2 teaspoons dried sage leaves, crushed

1/2 teaspoon ground black pepper

3 (3 1/2 x 6 1/4-inch) thin slices prosciutto or ham

1/4 teaspoon salt

1/4 teaspoon paprika

1/4 cup dry vermouth or white wine

3/4 cup chicken bouillon or broth

1 tablespoon all-purpose flour

2 tablespoons water

Cooked rice

Pound turkey cutlets between plastic wrap to about 1/4-inch thickness; set aside. Drain spinach; press out excess moisture with back of a large spoon. Combine spinach, parsley, bread crumbs, Parmesan cheese, pine nuts, 1 teaspoon of the sage, and 1/4 teaspoon pepper; mix well.

Halve prosciutto lengthwise. Place a half slice on each cutlet. Spoon about 1/2 cup spinach mixture on each. Starting at short end, roll up. Place in a 3 1/2-quart slow cooker, seam side down. Sprinkle each with salt, remaining 1/4 teaspoon pepper, and paprika. Pour vermouth or wine and bouillon around turkey rolls. Cover and cook on LOW 4 to 6 hours or until turkey is tender.

Remove turkey from slow cooker and keep warm. Turn control to HIGH. Add remaining teaspoon sage. In a small bowl, dissolve flour in water and add to slow cooker. Cook, stirring, on HIGH 10 to 15 minutes or until thickened. Slice each turkey roll and serve on cooked rice, topped with sauce.

Per serving without rice: Cal 113 · Carb 7 gm · Prot 29 gm · Total fat 3 gm · Sat fat 1 gm · Cal from fat 27 · Chol 68 mg · Sodium 503 mg

MALAYSIAN TURKEY CUTLETS

*B*uying a package of turkey breast cutlets or slices is a shortcut to an intriguing flavor combination highlighted by mint.

MAKES 5 OR 6 SERVINGS

1 cup fresh cilantro leaves

1/3 cup fresh mint leaves

2 tablespoons soy sauce

1 tablespoon vegetable oil

1/2 teaspoon chili oil

1 clove garlic, crushed

1 pound turkey breast cutlets

Process cilantro, mint, soy sauce, vegetable oil, chili oil, and garlic in a food processor until finely chopped. Brush on all sides of turkey and place in a 3 1/2-quart slow cooker. Pour any remaining sauce over turkey. Cover and cook on LOW about 4 hours or until turkey is tender.

Per serving: Cal 73 · Carb 2 gm · Prot 29 gm · Total fat 4 gm · Sat fat 1 gm · Cal from fat 36 · Chol 72 mg · Sodium 493 mg

TURKEY TOSTADA CRISPS

A topping of shredded jicama provides a pleasant crispy texture and flavor contrast.

MAKES 6 SERVINGS

1 medium onion, finely chopped

1 medium yellow bell pepper, seeded and chopped

1 large tomato, seeded and chopped

1/2 pound uncooked turkey breast, diced

1/2 teaspoon salt

1 (4-oz.) can diced green chiles, drained

1 (1.62-oz.) package spices and seasonings for enchilada
   sauce

1 tablespoon vegetable oil

6 (7-inch) flour tortillas

1/4 cup shredded Monterey Jack cheese

1 medium jicama, peeled and shredded

Combine onion, bell pepper, tomato, turkey, salt, green chiles, and seasoning mix in a 3 1/2-quart slow cooker. Cover and cook on LOW about 5 hours or until turkey and vegetables are tender.

Heat oil in a medium skillet. Add tortillas, one at a time, and cook until lightly browned on both sides and crispy. Spoon sauce on crisp tortillas. Top each with cheese and jicama.

Per serving: Cal 179 · Carb 24 gm · Prot 16 gm · Total fat 6 gm ·
Sat fat 1 gm · Cal from fat 54 · Chol 34 mg · Sodium 338 mg

FIVE-SPICE TURKEY THIGHS

*F*ive spice is a reddish-brown powder usually made of ground star anise, cloves, cinnamon, fennel, and Szechwan peppercorns.

MAKES ABOUT 6 SERVINGS

1 1/2 to 1 3/4 pounds boneless, skinless turkey thighs

2 green onions, including tops, minced

2 tablespoons soy sauce

2 tablespoons sherry

1 tablespoon sugar

1 teaspoon five-spice powder

1 teaspoon sesame oil

1/4 teaspoon ground black pepper

1 1/2 tablespoons cornstarch

2 tablespoons cold water

1 tablespoon sesame seeds, toasted (see Note, page 55)

1 tablespoon thin, diagonally sliced green onions

Hot cooked rice

Trim thighs of excess fat; tuck ends under to make a bundle. Place in a 3 1/2-quart slow cooker. Combine minced onions, soy sauce, sherry, sugar, five-spice powder, sesame oil, and pepper; mix well. Pour over turkey thighs. Cover and cook on LOW about 6 hours or until turkey is tender. Remove turkey from slow cooker and keep warm. Combine cornstarch and water until smooth and stir into cooking juices in slow cooker. Cover and cook on HIGH 15 to 20 minutes or until slightly thickened. Slice turkey; sprinkle with sesame seeds and sliced onions. Serve with rice and sauce.

Per serving: Cal 82 · Carb 5 gm · Prot 7 gm · Total fat 3 gm · Sat fat 0.5 gm · Cal from fat 27 · Chol 23 mg · Sodium 369 mg

TURKEY, YAM, AND APPLE STEW

*T*urkey breast can be substituted for the thighs in this slightly sweet dish.

MAKES ABOUT 6 SERVINGS

3/4 pound boneless, skinless turkey thighs, cut into bite-
size pieces

2 medium green apples, cored and diced

2 pounds yams, peeled and cut into 1-inch chunks

1/4 cup diced onion

1 cup chicken broth or bouillon

1/2 cup apple juice

2 tablespoons quick-cooking tapioca

1 tablespoon maple-flavored syrup

1/2 teaspoon ground cinnamon

1/2 teaspoon poultry seasoning

1/4 teaspoon salt

1/4 teaspoon ground white pepper

1/2 cup light sour cream or plain nonfat yogurt

Combine all ingredients, except sour cream or yogurt, in a 3 1/2-quart slow cooker. Cover and cook on LOW 6 to 7 hours or until yams are tender.

Serve in bowls with a dollop of light sour cream or plain non-fat yogurt.

Per serving: Cal 274 · Carb 58 gm · Prot 7 gm · Total fat 2 gm · Sat fat 0.5 gm · Cal from fat 18 · Chol 12 mg · Sodium 172 mg

TARRAGON-MUSTARD TURKEY
WITH FETTUCCINE

*I*f turkey is not available, substitute uncooked chicken.

MAKES 4 TO 6 SERVINGS

1 pound boneless, skinless turkey breast

2 leeks

2 stalks celery, chopped

1 tablespoon chopped fresh tarragon

2 tablespoons Dijon mustard

1 tablespoon fresh lemon juice

1 tablespoon brown sugar

1 teaspoon instant chicken bouillon granules

1/4 teaspoon salt

1/8 teaspoon ground black pepper

2 tablespoons cornstarch

2 tablespoons cold water

6 to 8 ounces fettuccine or medium pasta shells

Cut turkey into thin strips, about 1 x 1/4 inches. Trim leeks; halve lengthwise. Rinse and slice. Combine turkey and leeks in a 3 1/2-quart slow cooker with celery.

In a small bowl, combine tarragon, mustard, lemon juice, brown sugar, bouillon granules, salt, and pepper. Spoon over turkey. Cover and cook on LOW 4 1/2 to 5 hours or until turkey and vegetables are tender.

Turn control to HIGH. Dissolve cornstarch in cold water in a small bowl. Stir into cooking juices in slow cooker. Cover and cook on HIGH 20 to 30 minutes or until thickened.

Cook pasta according to package directions and drain. Spoon turkey mixture over cooked pasta.

Per serving: Cal 271 · Carb 48 gm · Prot 41 gm · Total fat 1 gm · Sat fat 0 gm · Cal from fat 9 · Chol 90 mg · Sodium 280 mg

PASTA WITH EASY
TURKEY-VEGETABLE SAUCE

*D*ouble the recipe and freeze half of mixture for another time.

MAKES 5 OR 6 SERVINGS

1 green bell pepper, diced

1 red onion, thinly sliced

8 to 10 ounces uncooked turkey breast, cut into strips

1 (14 1/2-oz.) jar chunky pizza sauce

3 small plum tomatoes, seeded and chopped

1/2 teaspoon dried oregano leaves

1 tablespoon chopped fresh basil, plus additional for
   garnish

1/4 teaspoon ground black pepper

8 ounces medium pasta shells or fettuccine

About 1 cup (4 ounces) shredded light mozzarella cheese

Combine bell pepper, onion, turkey, pizza sauce, tomatoes, oregano, basil, and black pepper in a 3 1/2-quart slow cooker. Cover and cook on LOW 5 to 6 hours or until turkey and vegetables are tender.

Cook pasta according to package directions and drain. Spoon sauce over cooked pasta. Top with cheese and additional basil.

Per serving: Cal 288 · Carb 44 gm · Prot 27 gm · Total fat 5 gm ·
Sat fat 3 gm · Cal from fat 45 · Chol 49 mg · Sodium 187 mg

MY FAVORITE PASTA SAUCE

*B*y using lean ground turkey and lean beef, you cut the cholesterol and calorie count, while creating an appealing flavor combination. Serve over cooked pasta or rice

MAKES ABOUT 6 SERVINGS

1/2 pound lean ground turkey

1/2 pound lean ground beef

1 stalk celery, chopped

2 medium carrots, peeled and chopped

1 clove garlic, crushed

1 medium onion, chopped

1 (28-oz.) can diced tomatoes with juice

1 (6-oz.) can tomato paste

1/2 teaspoon salt

1/8 teaspoon ground black pepper

1/4 teaspoon dried thyme

Combine ground turkey, beef, celery, carrots, garlic, and onion in a 3 1/2-quart slow cooker. Stir in diced tomatoes, tomato paste, salt, pepper, and thyme. Cover and cook on LOW 7 to 8 hours or until meat and vegetables are tender.

Per serving: Cal 212 · Carb 15 gm · Prot 16 gm · Total fat 10 gm · Sat fat 1 gm · Cal from fat 90 · Chol 56 mg · Sodium 487 mg

CHUNKY SPAGHETTI 'N' TURKEY MEATBALLS

*T*urkey-flavored sausage plus fresh herbs add texture and flavor to this spaghetti recipe.

MAKES 6 SERVINGS

1 medium onion, chopped

1 carrot, peeled and chopped

2 stalks celery, chopped

1 clove garlic, crushed

1 (8-oz.) can tomato sauce

1 tablespoon chopped fresh basil

2 teaspoons chopped fresh oregano

1 teaspoon chopped fresh thyme

1 teaspoon Worcestershire sauce

1/8 teaspoon ground black pepper

1 (28-oz.) can diced tomatoes with juice

1/2 pound mild Italian turkey sausage

1/2 pound extra-lean ground beef

1/3 cup seasoned dry bread crumbs

1 egg, beaten slightly

2 tablespoons milk

1 pound spaghetti, cooked and drained

Grated Parmesan cheese (optional)

Combine onion, carrot, celery, garlic, tomato sauce, basil, oregano, thyme, Worcestershire sauce, pepper, and tomatoes in a 3 1/2-quart slow cooker.

In a medium bowl, combine turkey sausage, ground beef, bread crumbs, egg, and milk. Form mixture into about 18 meatballs. Carefully place meatballs in sauce in slow cooker. Cover and cook on LOW about 7 hours or until meat and vegetables are tender.

Cook spaghetti according to package directions and drain. Spoon meatball mixture over cooked spaghetti. Sprinkle with grated Parmesan cheese, if desired.

Per serving: Cal 803 · Carb 145 gm · Prot 37 gm · Total fat 14 gm · Sat fat 1 gm · Cal from fat 126 · Chol 82 mg · Sodium 3638 mg

SOUTH-OF-THE-BORDER LASAGNA

*U*se turkey sausage and low-fat ricotta cheese to produce lasagna with lower fat and fewer calories.

MAKES 7 OR 8 SERVINGS

3/4 pound turkey sausage

2 tomatoes, seeded and chopped

3 fresh tomatillos, husked and chopped

1 (19-oz.) can green enchilada sauce

1 clove garlic, crushed

1/4 teaspoon salt

1/8 teaspoon ground black pepper

8 ounces lasagna noodles

1 cup low-fat or nonfat ricotta cheese

1 cup shredded reduced-fat jalapeño Jack cheese

Chopped fresh cilantro

Crumble sausage into a slow cooker. Stir in tomatoes, tomatillos, enchilada sauce, garlic, salt, and pepper. Cover and cook on LOW 5 1/2 to 6 hours.

Preheat oven to 350F (175C). Grease a 13 x 9-inch baking dish. Cook lasagna noodles according to package directions and drain. Spread about 1/2 cup turkey mixture in bottom of prepared pan; arrange alternate layers of noodles, ricotta cheese, and hot turkey mixture. Top with Jack cheese. Bake 25 to 30 minutes or until bubbly around edges. Sprinkle with cilantro.

Per serving: Cal 340 · Carb 36 gm · Prot 21 gm · Total fat 13 gm · Sat fat 3 gm · Cal from fat 117 · Chol 56 mg · Sodium 817 mg

TASTE-OF-THE-SOUTHWEST TURKEY LOAF

*V*arious combinations of fresh salsa are usually found in the deli case of your supermarket.

MAKES 5 OR 6 SERVINGS

1/2 cup refrigerated fresh salsa

2 tablespoons chopped fresh cilantro

1 green onion, including top, chopped

1 egg, slightly beaten

1/4 teaspoon ground cumin

1/4 teaspoon salt

1 zucchini, shredded

1 1/4 pounds ground turkey or chicken

In a medium bowl, combine salsa, cilantro, green onion, egg, cumin, salt, zucchini, and turkey. Form into a 6-inch-round loaf. Place loaf on a trivet in a 3 1/2-quart slow cooker. Cover and cook on LOW 4 to 4 1/2 hours.

Remove loaf from slow cooker. Cut into wedges and serve.

Per serving: Cal 199 · Carb 4 gm · Prot 21 gm · Total fat 10 gm · Sat fat 3 gm · Cal from fat 90 · Chol 134 mg · Sodium 404 mg

ROUND SESAME TURKEY LOAF

*T*he uncooked mixture will be fairly soft, but it will become firmer as it cooks.

MAKES 5 OR 6 SERVINGS

1 pound ground turkey

1 egg, slightly beaten

2 green onions, including some tops, chopped

2 tablespoons soy sauce

1/2 teaspoon grated gingerroot

1/4 cup chopped water chestnuts

2 tablespoons prepared sweet-and-sour sauce

1 cup cooked rice

1 tablespoon sesame seeds, toasted (see Note, page 55)

In a medium bowl, combine all ingredients except sesame seeds. Form into a 6-inch-round loaf. Press sesame seeds into top. Place loaf in a 3 1/2-quart slow cooker. Cover and cook on LOW about 4 hours.

Remove loaf from slow cooker. Cut into wedges and serve.

Per serving: Cal 228 · Carb 15 gm · Prot 18 gm · Total fat 9 gm · Sat fat 2 gm · Cal from fat 81 · Chol 115 mg · Sodium 530 mg

TERIYAKI TURKEY LOAF

*F*lavors of the Far East enhance this more traditional turkey loaf.

MAKES ABOUT 6 SERVINGS

1 1/4 pounds ground turkey

1/4 cup fine dry bread crumbs

1 egg, beaten slightly

1/2 cup finely chopped celery

2 green onions, including some tops, finely chopped

1/4 teaspoon salt

1/8 teaspoon ground black pepper

1/4 cup finely chopped green bell pepper

1/2 cup teriyaki sauce

1 (8-oz.) can sliced water chestnuts, drained

In a medium bowl, combine turkey, bread crumbs, egg, celery, green onions, salt, and black pepper. Form into a 5 1/2- to 6-inch-round loaf. Place loaf in a 3 1/2-quart slow cooker.

In a small bowl, combine bell pepper, teriyaki sauce, and water chestnuts. Spoon over loaf. Cover and cook on low about 4 hours.

Remove loaf from slow cooker. Cut into thin wedges or slices.

Per serving: Cal 186 · Carb 7 gm · Prot 18 gm · Total fat 9 gm · Sat fat 2 gm · Cal from fat 81 · Chol 111 mg · Sodium 628 mg

87

RASPBERRY-GLAZED TURKEY MEATBALLS

*Y*our friends will love this sweet-sour sauce with its intriguing raspberry flavor.

MAKES ABOUT 45 MEATBALLS

1/2 cup seedless raspberry fruit spread or preserves

2 tablespoons raspberry vinegar

2 tablespoons chili sauce

1/2 teaspoon ground cardamom

3/4 teaspoon salt

3/8 teaspoon ground black pepper

1 1/4 pounds lean ground turkey

1/3 cup quick-cooking oats

1/4 cup minced onion

1 large egg, slightly beaten

1 tablespoon Worcestershire sauce

1 teaspoon cornstarch

1 tablespoon cold water

Minced green onion

In a small bowl, whisk raspberry spread, vinegar, chili sauce, cardamom, 1/4 teaspoon salt, and 1/8 teaspoon pepper. Spread 3 tablespoons of mixture over bottom of a slow cooker; set remainder aside.

In a medium bowl, combine turkey, oats, onion, egg, Worcestershire sauce, remaining 1/2 teaspoon salt, and remaining 1/4 tea-

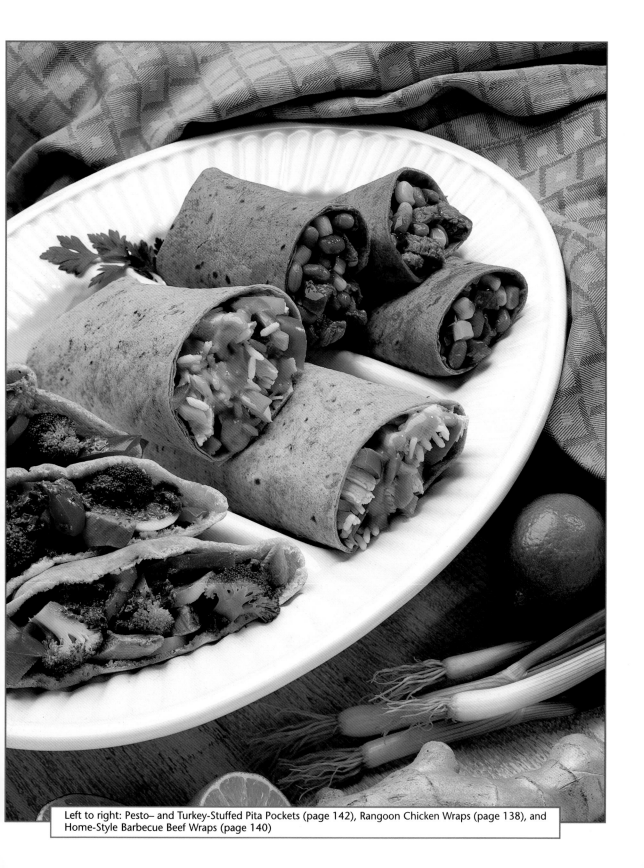

Left to right: Pesto– and Turkey-Stuffed Pita Pockets (page 142), Rangoon Chicken Wraps (page 138), and Home-Style Barbecue Beef Wraps (page 140)

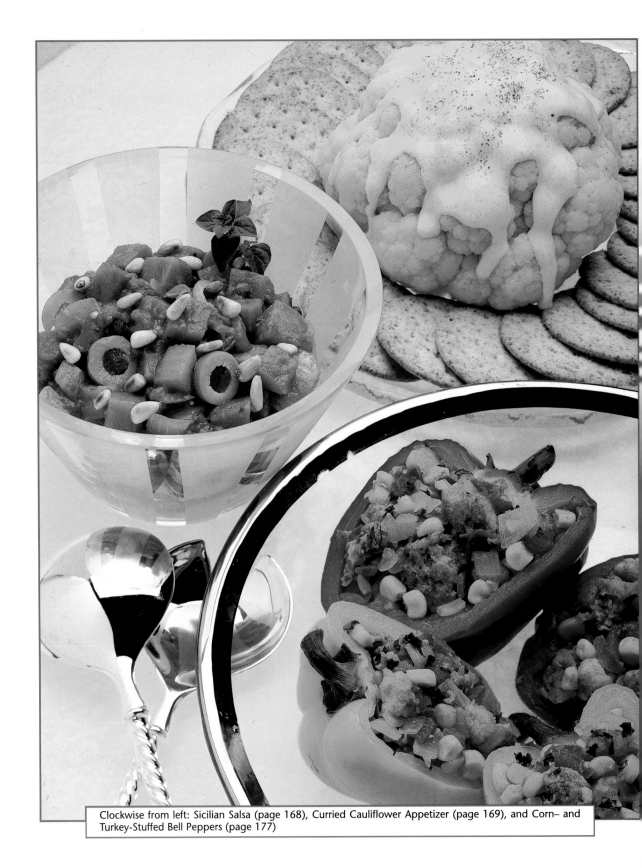

Clockwise from left: Sicilian Salsa (page 168), Curried Cauliflower Appetizer (page 169), and Corn– and Turkey-Stuffed Bell Peppers (page 177)

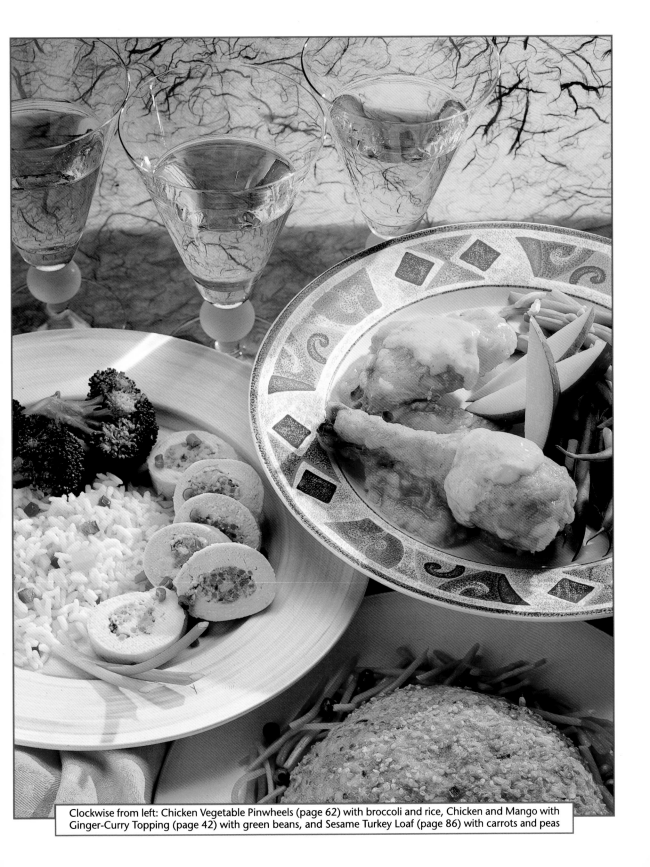

Clockwise from left: Chicken Vegetable Pinwheels (page 62) with broccoli and rice, Chicken and Mango with Ginger-Curry Topping (page 42) with green beans, and Sesame Turkey Loaf (page 86) with carrots and peas

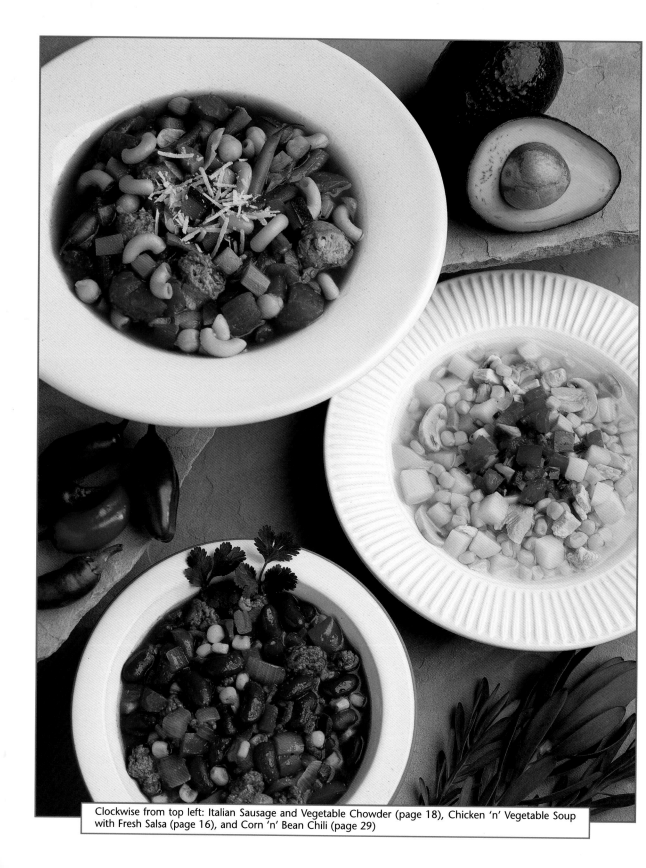

Clockwise from top left: Italian Sausage and Vegetable Chowder (page 18), Chicken 'n' Vegetable Soup with Fresh Salsa (page 16), and Corn 'n' Bean Chili (page 29)

spoon pepper. Shape into 1- to 1 1/2-inch balls. Place in sauce in slow cooker. Spoon remaining sauce over meatballs. Cover and cook on LOW 6 hours.

Turn control to HIGH. In a small bowl, dissolve cornstarch in water. Spoon over meatballs. Cover and cook on HIGH 5 to 10 minutes or until thickened. Sprinkle with green onions.

Per meatball: Cal 30 · Carb 2 gm · Prot 3 gm · Total fat 1 gm · Sat fat 0 gm · Cal from fat 9 · Chol 15 mg · Sodium 64 mg

TURKEY PORCUPINES IN ENCHILADA SAUCE

*T*he popular meat and rice meatballs turn Mexican and spicy!

MAKES 19 MEATBALLS OR 4 OR 5 SERVINGS

1 1/4 pounds lean ground turkey

1/2 cup white long-grain rice

1/2 cup finely chopped green bell pepper

2 tablespoons minced onion

1/2 teaspoon salt

1/4 teaspoon ground black pepper

1 (19-oz.) can enchilada sauce

1/4 cup water

In a medium bowl, combine turkey, rice, bell pepper, onion, salt, and black pepper; mix well. Shape mixture into balls about 1 1/2 inches in diameter; place in slow cooker. Combine enchilada sauce and water; pour over meatballs. Cover and cook on LOW about 6 hours or until rice is tender. To serve, spoon sauce over meatballs.

Per meatball: Cal 70 · Carb 5 gm · Prot 5 gm · Total fat 3 gm · Sat fat 1 gm · Cal from fat 27 · Chol 24 mg · Sodium 231 mg

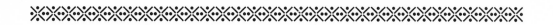

WELCOME WAYS WITH BEEF

*B*eef has always been one of the most popular meats to use in the slow cooker. It is so handy to be able to purchase a thrifty cut of beef, combine it with the appropriate seasonings, and then have a very flavorful meat dish ready to take out of the pot at dinnertime.

You can stretch your budget by watching for weekly specials on beef cuts that are offered at reduced prices for a limited time. If you can't use all the meat right away, freeze it and bring it out at a later date.

Remember that beef dishes prepared in a slow cooker result in more cooking juices than those made by other methods of cooking. Take advantage of these flavorful juices. At the end of cooking time remove the cooked beef from the slow cooker. Turn the control to HIGH and stir in cornstarch that is dissolved in cold water or bouillon. Cook 25 to 30 minutes; it will be transformed into a delicious sauce to spoon over the meat and vegetables.

Cooking Tip

An easy way to test a roast or meat loaf for doneness is to use an instant-read thermometer. Ground beef should be cooked to an internal temperature of 160F (72C) and a roast should be cooked to between 145 to 170F (65 to 75C), depending on desired doneness.

JICAMA-CILANTRO ROUND STEAK

*F*lavors will be more intense if you prepare the jicama mixture the day before and refrigerate it until serving time.

MAKES 5 OR 6 SERVINGS

1 to 1 1/4 pounds boneless beef round steak

1 tablespoon instant beef bouillon granules

1/8 teaspoon ground black pepper

1 large tomato, chopped

1 small jicama, peeled and coarsely shredded

2 tablespoons chopped fresh cilantro

2 green onions, including some tops, chopped

1 teaspoon grated gingerroot

1 small jalapeño chile, seeded and finely chopped

1 teaspoon vegetable oil

Trim and discard fat from steak; cut into 5 or 6 pieces. Place steak in a 3 1/2-quart slow cooker. Sprinkle with bouillon granules and pepper. Top with tomato. Cover and cook on LOW 7 to 8 hours or until steak is tender.

While meat cooks, combine jicama, cilantro, green onions, ginger, jalapeño chile, and oil in a small bowl and refrigerate.

Remove steak from slow cooker. Spoon jicama mixture over each serving.

Per serving: Cal 210 · Carb 3 gm · Prot 19 gm · Total fat 13 gm · Sat fat 5 gm · Cal from fat 117 · Chol 55 mg · Sodium 215 mg

CREOLE BEEF AND PEPPER STRIPS WITH CURLY NOODLES

*T*his is a popular and tasty way to make a small amount of meat serve more people.

MAKES 5 OR 6 SERVINGS

3/4 pound boneless beef round steak

1 green or red bell pepper, chopped

1 medium onion, chopped

1 clove garlic, crushed

1 medium tomato, chopped

1 beef bouillon cube

1/2 cup boiling water

1 tablespoon chopped parsley

1/2 teaspoon chopped fresh thyme

1/2 teaspoon salt

1/8 teaspoon ground black pepper

2 tablespoons cornstarch

2 tablespoons cold water

6 ounces curly noodles

Slice steak into diagonal strips about 1/4 inch thick. Combine steak, pepper, onion, garlic, and tomato in a 3 1/2-quart slow cooker. Dissolve bouillon cube in boiling water. Add to slow cooker with parsley, thyme, salt, and pepper. Cover and cook on LOW about 7 hours or until steak is tender.

Turn control to HIGH. In a small bowl, dissolve cornstarch in cold water. Stir into slow cooker. Cover and cook on HIGH about 10 minutes or until slightly thickened.

Meanwhile, cook noodles according to package directions and drain. Spoon steak mixture over noodles.

Per serving: Cal 289 · Carb 31 gm · Prot 19 gm · Total fat 10 gm · Sat fat 4 gm · Cal from fat 90 · Chol 41 mg · Sodium 409 mg

NEW-STYLE BEEF STROGANOFF

*R*educed-fat sour cream cuts the calories and fats, yet provides the traditional stroganoff flavor.

MAKES 6 TO 8 SERVINGS

1 1/2 to 1 3/4 pounds boneless beef round steak

1 onion, sliced

1 clove garlic, crushed

1 tablespoon Worcestershire sauce

1/4 teaspoon ground black pepper

1/4 teaspoon salt

1/2 teaspoon paprika

1 (10 1/2-oz.) can condensed beef broth

2 tablespoons ketchup

1 tablespoon red wine

3 tablespoons cornstarch

1/4 cup cold water

1/4 pound fresh mushrooms, sliced

3/4 cup reduced-fat sour cream

Trim all visible fat from steak. Cut steak into 1/4-inch-thick slices. Place steak in a 3 1/2-quart slow cooker. Add onion, garlic, Worcestershire sauce, pepper, salt, paprika, broth, ketchup, and wine. Cover and cook on LOW 6 to 8 hours or until steak is tender. Turn control to HIGH. Dissolve cornstarch in water. Add to slow cooker. Stir in mushrooms. Cover and cook 15 to 30 minutes or until bubbly. Stir in sour cream and serve.

Per serving: Cal 400 · Carb 21 gm · Prot 33 gm · Total fat 20 gm · Sat fat 6 gm · Cal from fat 180 · Chol 75 mg · Sodium 390 mg

TASTE-OF-ACAPULCO FLANK STEAK

*T*he combination of tomatillos and baby corn gives the steak a distinctive yet pleasant flavor.

MAKES 6 OR 7 SERVINGS

1 (1 1/2- to 2-lb.) beef flank steak

6 fresh tomatillos

1 (15-oz.) can whole baby corn-on-the-cob, drained

1/2 teaspoon salt

1/4 teaspoon ground black pepper

1/4 cup chopped fresh cilantro

1 small red onion, thinly sliced

1/4 cup dry red wine

Trim all visible fat from steak. Place steak in a 3 1/2-quart slow cooker. Remove and discard husk and stem from tomatillos; chop and add to steak. Top with baby corn, salt, pepper, cilantro, and onion. Pour in wine. Cover and cook on LOW about 6 hours or until steak is tender.

Slice steak crosswise into strips; spoon vegetables and sauce over sliced steak.

Per serving: Cal 245 · Carb 14 gm · Prot 26 gm · Total fat 9 gm · Sat fat 4 gm · Cal from fat 81 · Chol 56 mg · Sodium 283 mg

THREE-PEPPER STEAK

A colorful array of peppers combined with onions and tomatoes yield an appetizing main dish.

MAKES 5 OR 6 SERVINGS

1 (1- to 1 1/4-lb.) beef flank steak

1 yellow bell pepper

1 green bell pepper

1/4 teaspoon salt

1/2 teaspoon red pepper flakes

3 green onions, including some tops, chopped

2 tablespoons soy sauce

2 medium tomatoes, chopped

Trim all visible fat from steak. Place steak in a 3 1/2-quart slow cooker. Remove stems and seeds from yellow and green peppers; cut into strips. Arrange bell peppers on steak. Sprinkle with salt. Top with red pepper flakes, green onions, soy sauce, and tomatoes. Cover and cook on LOW 6 to 7 hours or until steak is tender.

Per serving: Cal 163 · Carb 5 gm · Prot 21 gm · Total fat 7 gm · Sat fat 3 gm · Cal from fat 63 · Chol 45 mg · Sodium 590 mg

BARBECUED BRISKET 'N' NOODLES

*K*eep the calories as low as possible by selecting the leanest brisket and trimming off excess fat.

MAKES 8 TO 10 SERVINGS

1 (2- to 2 1/2-lb.) flat-cut beef brisket

1 cup bottled hickory-smoke barbecue sauce

1 tablespoon prepared horseradish

1 teaspoon prepared mustard

1/4 teaspoon salt

1/8 teaspoon ground black pepper

12 ounces wide noodles

Place brisket in a 3 1/2-quart slow cooker. In a small bowl, combine barbecue sauce, horseradish, mustard, salt, and pepper. Pour over brisket. Cover and cook on LOW 7 to 8 hours or until brisket is tender.

Cook noodles according to package directions; drain. Slice meat. Arrange sliced meat on noodles and top with sauce.

Per serving: Cal 514 · Carb 36 gm · Prot 26 gm · Total fat 28 gm · Sat fat 11 gm · Cal from fat 252 · Chol 80 mg · Sodium 410 mg

POT ROAST WITH AVOCADO-CHILE TOPPING

*T*he topping adds a fresh flavor to a traditional pot roast.

MAKES 8 TO 10 SERVINGS

1 (3- to 3 1/2-lb.) boneless lean beef pot roast

1/4 teaspoon salt

1/8 teaspoon ground black pepper

1/8 teaspoon garlic salt

1 large onion, sliced

1 small ripe avocado

2 tablespoons minced fresh cilantro

1 teaspoon fresh lemon juice

1 (4-oz.) can chopped green chiles, drained

1 teaspoon Worcestershire sauce

1/2 teaspoon prepared horseradish

Sprinkle roast with salt, pepper, and garlic salt. Place in a 3 1/2-quart slow cooker. Top with sliced onion. Cover and cook on LOW 8 to 9 hours or until roast is tender. While roast is cooking, peel, pit, and mash avocado. Combine avocado, cilantro, lemon juice, chiles, Worcestershire sauce, and horseradish in a medium bowl. Cover and refrigerate.

Remove roast from slow cooker and slice. Arrange sliced roast on individual plates. Spoon onion and cooking juices over each serving and top with a dollop of avocado mixture.

Per serving: Cal 400 · Carb 5 gm · Prot 35 gm · Total fat 26 gm · Sat fat 9 gm · Cal from fat 234 · Chol 103 mg · Sodium 210 mg

MOROCCAN-STYLE POT ROAST WITH COUSCOUS

*T*he spices of this one-pot meal are reminiscent of those used in Morocco.

MAKES 7 OR 8 SERVINGS

1 teaspoon ground ginger

1/2 teaspoon turmeric

1/4 teaspoon ground cumin

1/2 teaspoon paprika

1/2 teaspoon salt

1/4 teaspoon ground black pepper

1 (3- to 4-lb.) boneless lean beef pot roast

1 medium onion

7 or 8 parsnips

1 (10-oz.) package couscous

In a small bowl, combine ginger, turmeric, cumin, paprika, salt, and pepper. Press into both sides of roast. Let stand while preparing vegetables. Slice onion; place on bottom of a 4- or 5-quart slow cooker. Peel parsnips and cut into 2-inch lengths. Place spiced beef on onion; top with parsnips. Cover and cook on LOW 7 to 8 hours or until roast is tender.

Prepare couscous according to package directions. Serve couscous with pot roast and vegetables.

Per serving: Cal 623 · Carb 48 gm · Prot 45 gm · Total fat 26 gm · Sat fat 10 gm · Cal from fat 237 · Chol 118 mg · Sodium 262 mg

POT ROAST WITH BASIL, SUN-DRIED TOMATOES, AND PINE NUTS

*P*opular pesto ingredients are combined to produce a favorite pot roast.

MAKES ABOUT 8 SERVINGS

1/3 cup dry-packed sun-dried tomatoes

1/2 cup boiling water

1 clove garlic, chopped

1 (2 1/2- to 3-lb.) boneless beef round or pot roast

1 medium onion, sliced

2 tablespoons chopped fresh basil

1/4 teaspoon salt

1/8 teaspoon ground black pepper

2 tablespoons chopped pine nuts, toasted (see Note, page 165)

Combine tomatoes and boiling water in a medium bowl. Add garlic; let stand about 5 minutes.

Place roast in a 3 1/2-quart slow cooker. Top with onion, basil, salt, and pepper. Pour tomato mixture over all. Cover and cook on LOW about 8 hours or until roast is tender.

Remove roast to a serving dish. Sprinkle with pine nuts. Serve with tomato drippings, if desired.

Per serving: Cal 315 · Carb 3 gm · Prot 29 gm · Total fat 20 gm · Sat fat 7 gm · Cal from fat 180 · Chol 86 mg · Sodium 143 mg

SHORTCUT CHUCK ROAST
WITH MUSHROOM SAUCE

*F*or even lower fat content, cook this recipe the day before you want to serve it. Refrigerate overnight; remove fat from surface and reheat the dish before serving.

MAKES 6 OR 7 SERVINGS

1 (2- to 2 1/2-lb.) boneless beef chuck roast

1 (1-oz.) envelope dry onion soup mix

1 (10 3/4-oz.) can reduced-fat condensed cream of
mushroom soup

8 to 10 fresh mushrooms, sliced

Trim and discard visible fat from all sides of roast. Place roast in a 3 1/2-quart slow cooker. In a small bowl, combine dry soup mix with condensed soup. Pour over roast. Add mushrooms. Cover and cook on LOW 6 to 8 hours or until roast is tender.

Remove roast from slow cooker and slice. Serve with cooking juices.

Per serving: Cal 466 · Carb 7 gm · Prot 30 gm · Total fat 33 gm ·
Sat fat 13 gm · Cal from fat 297 · Chol 103 mg · Sodium 925 mg

NAVAJO BEEF AND CHILE STEW

If you don't care for spicy food, reduce the amount of ground red pepper to 1/8 teaspoon.

MAKES ABOUT 4 SERVINGS

3/4 pound lean beef stew meat, cut into 3/4-inch cubes

1 large onion, chopped

2 large cloves garlic, minced

1 (14 1/2-oz.) can ready-cut tomatoes with juice

1 (7-oz.) can diced green chiles, drained

1 (8.5-oz.) can whole-kernel corn, undrained

1 1/2 teaspoons dried oregano leaves, crushed

1 teaspoon ground cumin

1/2 teaspoon salt

1/4 teaspoon ground red pepper

2 tablespoons yellow cornmeal

Combine all ingredients, except cornmeal, in a 3 1/2-quart slow cooker, mixing well. Cover and cook on LOW 7 to 8 hours or until meat is tender.

Turn control to HIGH. Stir in cornmeal. Cover and cook on high 20 to 25 minutes.

Per serving: Cal 292 · Carb 27 gm · Prot 20 gm · Total fat 11 gm · Sat fat 4 gm · Cal from fat 99 · Chol 51 mg · Sodium 685 mg

GARDEN VEGETABLE–BEEF STEW

*F*or the best flavor, use fresh herbs and vegetables.

MAKES ABOUT 6 SERVINGS

3 medium potatoes, peeled and cut into eighths

4 medium carrots, peeled and cut into 1-inch pieces

1 leek, cut into 1/2-inch pieces and rinsed

1 pound lean beef stew meat, cut into 1-inch pieces

1 red or yellow bell pepper, cut into 1-inch pieces

2 cups fresh or frozen green beans

1 (14 1/2-oz.) can beef broth

2 tablespoons chopped fresh parsley

1 teaspoon chopped fresh marjoram

1 teaspoon chopped fresh oregano

1/2 teaspoon salt

1/8 teaspoon ground black pepper

2 teaspoons Worcestershire sauce

3 tablespoons cornstarch

3 tablespoons cold water

Place potatoes, carrots, and leek in a 3 1/2-quart slow cooker. Top with beef, bell pepper, and green beans. In a small bowl, combine beef broth with parsley, marjoram, oregano, salt, pepper, and Worcestershire sauce. Pour broth mixture over beef and vegetables. Cover and cook on LOW 8 to 10 hours or until beef is tender. Turn control to HIGH. In a small bowl, dissolve cornstarch in cold water and add to stew mixture. Cover and cook on HIGH about 20 minutes, stirring occasionally, until thickened.

Per serving: Cal 268 · Carb 26 gm · Prot 19 gm · Total fat 10 gm · Sat fat 4 gm · Cal from fat 90 · Chol 45 mg · Sodium 482 mg

SAUERBRATEN-STYLE SHORT RIBS

*U*se lean short ribs if available and scoop off any excess fat from the top of the sauce before adding gingersnaps.

MAKES ABOUT 6 SERVINGS

2 to 2 1/2 pounds beef short ribs

1/2 cup red wine

1 lemon, sliced

1 onion, sliced

5 peppercorns

10 whole cloves

1 tablespoon pickling spices

1/2 cup water

12 gingersnaps, crumbled

Place ribs in a large ceramic or glass bowl. In a small bowl, combine wine, lemon, onion, peppercorns, cloves, pickling spices, and water. Pour over short ribs. Cover and refrigerate overnight, turning ribs at least once during marinating.

Place marinated ribs in a 3 1/2-quart slow cooker. Pour marinade over ribs. Cover and cook on LOW about 8 hours or until ribs are tender. Remove ribs and keep warm. Strain juices and return to slow cooker. Turn control to HIGH. Stir in gingersnaps; cover and cook on HIGH about 15 minutes or until thickened. Spoon sauce over ribs.

Per serving: Cal 575 · Carb 12 gm · Prot 26 gm · Total fat 44 gm · Sat fat 17 gm · Cal from fat 396 · Chol 108 mg · Sodium 122 mg

ASPARAGUS CUBE STEAK ROLL-UPS

*A*n easy-to-put-together meal, the results are a meat and two vegetables from one pot.

MAKES 5 OR 6 SERVINGS

8 to 10 small new potatoes

5 or 6 (5- to 7-oz.) cube steaks

10 to 12 asparagus spears, trimmed

1 (0.75-oz.) package dry garlic and herb salad mix

Place potatoes in a 3 1/2-quart slow cooker. Top each cube steak with 2 asparagus spears. Roll up; secure with wooden picks if necessary. Place roll-ups, seam side down, over potatoes in slow cooker. Sprinkle dry salad mix over all. Cover and cook on LOW 5 1/2 to 6 hours or until meat is tender.

Per serving: Cal 436 · Carb 35 gm · Prot 33 gm · Total fat 19 gm · Sat fat 7 gm · Cal from fat 171 · Chol 85 mg · Sodium 634 mg

SUN-DRIED TOMATO MEAT LOAF

*A*dding sun-dried tomatoes and couscous to traditional meat loaf results in an interesting flavor and texture variation.

MAKES 6 OR 7 SERVINGS

1 cup boiling water

1/4 cup dry-packed sun-dried tomatoes

1 1/4 pounds lean ground beef

1/3 cup plain couscous

1 egg, slightly beaten

1/4 cup milk

1/4 cup chopped green bell pepper

2 green onions, including tops, chopped

1/4 teaspoon salt

1/8 teaspoon ground black pepper

1/2 teaspoon chili powder

Pour boiling water over sun-dried tomatoes. Cover and let stand 2 or 3 minutes or until softened. Drain; finely chop.

In a medium bowl, combine tomatoes with ground beef, couscous, egg, milk, bell pepper, green onions, salt, black pepper, and chili powder. Form into a 7 x 6-inch oval. Place on a trivet in a 3 1/2-quart slow cooker. Cover and cook on LOW 5 to 6 hours or until done.

Per serving: Cal 314 · Carb 9 gm · Prot 20 gm · Total fat 21 gm · Sat fat 8 gm · Cal from fat 189 · Chol 108 mg · Sodium 177 mg

CHILE AND CORN-CHIP MEAT LOAF

*C*rushed corn chips provide an interesting texture with a South-of-the-border flavor.

MAKES 5 OR 6 SERVINGS

1 cup corn chips

1 small green chile, seeded and finely chopped

2 tablespoons finely chopped fresh cilantro

1 teaspoon chili powder

1/2 teaspoon ground cumin

1/4 teaspoon salt

1 egg, slightly beaten

1 (8-oz.) can tomato sauce

1 pound lean ground beef

Crush corn chips until they are coarse crumbs. In a large bowl, combine corn chips, green chile, cilantro, chili powder, cumin, and salt. Stir in egg, half of the tomato sauce, and the ground beef. Form mixture into an 8-inch round loaf. Place loaf on a trivet in a 3 1/2-quart slow cooker. Spoon remaining tomato sauce over loaf. Cover and cook on LOW about 4 hours or until done.

Remove loaf and slice; spoon cooking juices over slices, if desired.

Per serving: Cal 300 · Carb 7 gm · Prot 18 gm · Total fat 21 gm · Sat fat 8 gm · Cal from fat 189 · Chol 110 mg · Sodium 477 mg

CONFETTI MEAT LOAF

*T*his interesting flavor combination will encourage everyone to enjoy vegetables with their meat.

MAKES 6 SERVINGS

1 pound lean ground beef

1/4 pound pork sausage

1 egg, slightly beaten

1/4 cup finely chopped leek

1/3 cup fine dry bread crumbs

2 tablespoons taco sauce

1/2 teaspoon salt

1/8 teaspoon ground black pepper

2 teaspoons chopped fresh basil

1 medium to large zucchini, shredded

1 medium carrot, shredded

In a large bowl, combine beef, sausage, egg, leek, bread crumbs, taco sauce, salt, pepper, basil, zucchini, and carrot. Form into a 5 1/2-inch flattened round loaf. Place loaf on a trivet in a 3 1/2-quart slow cooker. Cover and cook on LOW about 4 hours or until done.

Remove loaf and cut into 6 wedges; spoon cooking juices over each serving.

Per serving: Cal 285 · Carb 8 gm · Prot 18 gm · Total fat 20 gm · Sat fat 8 gm · Cal from fat 180 · Chol 100 mg · Sodium 431 mg

PORCUPINE MEATBALLS IN TOMATO SAUCE

*K*ids will love these tasty morsels and adults will enjoy being kids again.

MAKES 24 TO 26 MEATBALLS

2 (8-oz.) cans tomato sauce

1/4 teaspoon garlic powder

1/2 teaspoon ground thyme

1/2 cup water

1 1/4 pounds lean ground beef

1/2 cup long-grain rice

2 tablespoons minced onion

1/2 teaspoon salt

1/4 teaspoon ground black pepper

Combine tomato sauce, garlic powder, thyme, and water in a 3 1/2-quart slow cooker.

In a medium bowl, combine beef, rice, onion, salt, and pepper, mixing well. Shape into 24 to 26 balls about the size of golf balls. Place meatballs in tomato mixture in slow cooker. Cover and cook on LOW 7 to 8 hours or until rice is tender. Serve sauce over meatballs.

Per meatball: Cal 80 · Carb 4 gm · Prot 5 gm · Total fat 5 gm · Sat fat 2 gm · Cal from fat 45 · Chol 18 mg · Sodium 118 mg

MEATBALLS IN SUN-DRIED TOMATO GRAVY

*T*hese meatballs are best when served over cooked noodles, fettuccine, or spaghetti.

MAKES 6 OR 7 SERVINGS

1 cup boiling water

1/4 cup dry-packed sun-dried tomatoes

1 small onion, chopped

1 stalk celery, chopped

2 teaspoons chopped fresh basil

2 teaspoons chopped fresh oregano

1 tablespoon Worcestershire sauce

1 (10 1/2-oz.) can condensed beef broth

1/4 teaspoon salt

1/8 teaspoon ground black pepper

1 pound extra-lean ground beef

1/2 pound mild Italian turkey sausage

1/2 cup Italian-style dry bread crumbs

1 egg, slightly beaten

1/4 cup milk

3 tablespoons cornstarch

1/4 cup cold water

In a medium bowl, pour boiling water over tomatoes. Cover and let stand about 15 minutes or until softened. Drain; finely chop. Combine tomatoes, onion, celery, basil, oregano, Worcestershire sauce, beef broth, salt, and pepper in a 3 1/2-quart slow cooker.

In a medium bowl, combine beef, sausage, bread crumbs, egg, and milk, mixing well. Form into 20 to 22 meatballs about the size of golf balls. Place meatballs in tomato mixture in slow cooker. Cover and cook on LOW 4 to 5 hours or until vegetables are tender.

Turn control to HIGH. In a small bowl, dissolve cornstarch in cold water. Stir into slow cooker. Cover and cook on HIGH 15 to 20 minutes. Serve sauce over meatballs.

Per serving: Cal 356 · Carb 20 gm · Prot 25 gm · Total fat 18 gm · Sat fat 1 gm · Cal from fat 162 · Chol 110 mg · Sodium 880 mg

FIESTA TAMALE PIE

*C*hoose a mild or spicy salsa, depending on your family's preferences.

MAKES ABOUT 6 SERVINGS

3/4 cup yellow cornmeal

1 cup beef broth

1 pound extra-lean ground beef

1 teaspoon chili powder

1/2 teaspoon ground cumin

1 (14- to 16-oz.) jar thick and chunky salsa

1 (16-oz.) can whole-kernel corn, drained

1/4 cup sliced ripe olives

2 ounces reduced-fat Cheddar cheese, shredded

  (1/2 cup)

In a large bowl, mix cornmeal and broth; let stand 5 minutes. Stir in beef, chili powder, cumin, salsa, corn, and olives. Pour into a 3 1/2-quart slow cooker. Cover and cook on LOW 5 to 7 hours or until set.

Sprinkle cheese over top; cover and cook another 5 minutes or until cheese melts.

Per serving: Cal 350 · Carb 34 gm · Prot 21 gm · Total fat 16 gm · Sat fat 0 gm · Cal from fat 144 · Chol 57 mg · Sodium 935 mg

CABBAGE BURGER BAKE

*R*eminiscent of stuffed cabbage rolls, this dish is quicker to prepare when the cabbage is shredded and the spaghetti sauce is already prepared for you.

MAKES 6 SERVINGS

1 (1-lb.) package (about 6 cups) shredded cabbage and carrots

3/4 pound lean ground beef

1/2 teaspoon salt

1/4 teaspoon ground black pepper

1 medium onion, finely chopped

1 cup long-grain rice

1 (26-oz.) can chunky low-fat spaghetti sauce

1/2 cup water

1/4 teaspoon dried basil leaves, crushed

1/4 teaspoon seasoned salt

Place 1/2 of the cabbage and carrots in a 3 1/2-quart slow cooker. Crumble ground beef over top. Sprinkle with 1/4 teaspoon of the salt and 1/8 teaspoon of the pepper. Evenly distribute onion, then rice over all. Top with remaining cabbage, salt, and pepper. Combine spaghetti sauce, water, basil, and seasoned salt; pour over cabbage. Cover and cook on LOW 5 to 6 hours or until rice is tender.

Per serving: Cal 358 · Carb 42 gm · Prot 16 gm · Total fat 14 gm · Sat fat 5 gm · Cal from fat 126 · Chol 42 mg · Sodium 985 mg

EIGHT-LAYER CASSEROLE

*T*his many-layered but quick-to-assemble, stick-to-the-ribs casserole is perfect for a family meal.

MAKES 4 OR 5 SERVINGS

1/2 pound lean ground beef

2 tablespoons imitation bacon bits

1 small onion, chopped

1 (15-oz.) can tomato sauce

1/2 cup water

1/2 teaspoon chili powder

1/4 teaspoon salt

1/4 teaspoon ground black pepper

2/3 cup long-grain rice

1 (8 3/4-oz.) can whole-kernel corn, drained

1/2 cup chopped green bell pepper

Crumble ground beef evenly over bottom of a 3 1/2-quart slow cooker. Sprinkle with bacon bits, then onion. In a medium bowl, combine tomato sauce, water, chili powder, salt, and black pepper; pour half over beef and onion layers. Sprinkle rice evenly over top, then corn. Top with remaining tomato sauce mixture, then bell pepper. Cover and cook on LOW about 5 hours or until rice is tender.

Per serving: Cal 365 · Carb 47 gm · Prot 16 gm · Total fat 13 gm · Sat fat 5 gm · Cal from fat 117 · Chol 42 mg · Sodium 1071 mg

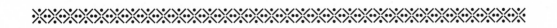

SATISFYING TASTES WITH PORK AND LAMB

*I*n the past, pork and lamb dishes were often heavily laden with calories and cholesterol. Today, we have the opportunity to purchase leaner cuts of these meats, because the animals are produced differently. Also, we have learned to trim and discard excess fat from roasts and chops before they are put into the slow cooker.

As a result, the cooked sauce in the slow cooker is a combination of natural meat juices and seasonings or your favorite vegetables. We have combined compatible flavors that enhance each specific kind of meat, such as a pork roast that is coated with lightly spiced cranberry sauce accented with candied ginger.

Cooking Tip

An easy way to test a roast or meat loaf for doneness is to use an instant-read thermometer. Ground pork and lamb should be cooked to an internal temperature of 160F (72C); a pork roast should be cooked to 160F (72C); and a lamb roast or chops to between 145 and 170F (65 and 75C), depending on desired doneness.

CRANBERRY-PORT PORK ROAST

*T*his hearty yet elegant dish is one of our favorites.

MAKES 6 TO 8 SERVINGS

1 (2 1/2- to 3-lb.) lean boneless pork loin roast

1 (16-oz.) can whole-berry cranberry sauce

1/3 cup port or cranberry juice

1/4 cup sugar

1/2 small lemon, thinly sliced

1/3 cup golden seedless raisins

1 large clove garlic, minced

2 tablespoons diced candied ginger

1/2 teaspoon dry mustard

1/2 teaspoon salt

1/4 teaspoon ground black pepper

3 tablespoons cornstarch

2 tablespoons cold water

Cooked rice

Place pork roast in a 3 1/2-quart slow cooker. In a medium bowl, combine cranberry sauce, port or juice, and sugar. Stir in lemon, raisins, garlic, ginger, mustard, salt, and pepper. Spoon over roast. Cover and cook on LOW 6 to 7 hours or until meat is 170F (75C) on an instant-read thermometer. Remove roast from slow cooker; cover with foil to keep it warm. Measure 3 cups of cooking juices and pour into a medium saucepan. Bring to a boil over medium-high heat. In a cup, dissolve cornstarch in cold water. Stir into saucepan. Cook, stirring, until thickened. Slice roast; serve with sauce and rice.

Per serving: Cal 514 · Carb 48 gm · Prot 35 gm · Total fat 18 gm ·
Sat fat 6 gm · Cal from fat 162 · Chol 98 mg · Sodium 275 mg

3C 4½P IF

PORK AND APPLE HOT-POT

*C*ut fairly thick slices of pork, then pass the sauce.

MAKES ABOUT 8 SERVINGS

1 (3 1/2- to 4-lb.) boneless pork shoulder roast

2 cooking apples, cored, peeled, and quartered

1 onion, thinly sliced

1 cup apple cider or juice

1 teaspoon chopped fresh thyme

1 teaspoon chopped fresh parsley

1/2 teaspoon seasoned salt

1/8 teaspoon ground black pepper

1 tablespoon brown sugar

3 tablespoons cornstarch

1/4 cup cold water

Place roast in a 4- to 6-quart slow cooker. Top with apples and onion; add cider or juice. Combine thyme, parsley, seasoned salt, pepper, and brown sugar; sprinkle over all. Cover and cook on LOW about 9 hours or until meat is 170F (75C) on an instant-read thermometer.

Remove roast, apples, and onion. Turn control to HIGH. In a small bowl, dissolve cornstarch in water. Add to juices in pot. Cover and cook, stirring occasionally, about 10 to 15 minutes or until slightly thickened. Slice roast; serve with sauce.

Per serving: Cal 543 · Carb 14 gm · Prot 35 gm · Total fat 37 gm · Sat fat 13 gm · Cal from fat 333 · Chol 145 mg · Sodium 221 mg

MUSTARDY ORANGE-FLAVORED PORK DINNER

A complete dinner in the slow cooker saves energy.

MAKES 8 SERVINGS

1 (6-oz.) can frozen orange juice concentrate, thawed

2 tablespoons Dijon mustard

1 teaspoon prepared horseradish

1 tablespoon honey

1 tablespoon grated onion

1/4 teaspoon salt

1/8 teaspoon ground black pepper

18 small white pearl onions, peeled

1 (4-lb.) lean pork butt roast with bone

3 medium sweet potatoes, peeled and quartered

1/4 cup cornstarch

Set aside about 6 tablespoons or half the orange juice concentrate. In a small bowl, combine remaining concentrate, mustard, horseradish, honey, grated onion, salt, and pepper. Place pearl onions in bottom of a 4-quart slow cooker. Trim and discard visible fat from pork and add to slow cooker. Arrange sweet potatoes around roast. Brush everything with mustard mixture. Cover and cook on LOW 8 to 9 hours or until meat is 170F (75C) on an instant-read thermometer. Remove roast, onions, and potatoes and cover with foil to keep warm. Dissolve cornstarch in reserved juice concentrate. Stir into cooking juices in slow cooker. Cover and cook on HIGH 15 to 20 minutes or until slightly thickened. Spoon over roast and vegetables.

Per serving: Cal 680 · Carb 29 gm · Prot 41 gm · Total fat 43 gm · Sat fat 14 gm · Cal from fat 387 · Chol 166 mg · Sodium 194 mg

121

PORK CHOPS WITH MINTED HERB RELISH

A refreshing, yet spicy combination of seasonings enhances the flavor of the pork chops.

MAKES 5 OR 6 SERVINGS

2 medium tomatoes, chopped

1 tablespoon chopped fresh basil

1 tablespoon chopped fresh mint

1 small jalapeño chile, seeded and finely chopped

2 teaspoons chopped fresh chives

2 teaspoons Dijon mustard

1 teaspoon prepared horseradish

1/8 teaspoon ground black pepper

1/4 teaspoon salt

5 or 6 pork chops or cutlets

In a small bowl, combine tomatoes, basil, mint, jalapeño chile, and chives. Cover and refrigerate.

In a small bowl, combine mustard, horseradish, salt, and pepper. Spread on one side of each pork chop. Place chops in a 3 1/2-quart slow cooker. Cover and cook on LOW about 4 hours or until meat is tender. Serve with chilled relish.

Per serving: Cal 200 · Carb 2 gm · Prot 21 gm · Total fat 11 gm · Sat fat 4 gm · Cal from fat 99 · Chol 59 mg · Sodium 172 mg

HARVEST PORK CHOPS

*W*hat could be more welcoming than coming home after an afternoon of shopping or errands to the delicious aroma of the spices in this dish!

MAKES 5 SERVINGS

5 boneless pork chops or cutlets (about 1 lb.)

1/8 teaspoon ground red pepper

1/2 teaspoon garlic salt

1 (1- to 1 1/4-lb.) Butternut or Delicata squash

2 medium oranges, peeled and sliced

1/4 teaspoon ground cinnamon

1/4 teaspoon ground cloves

1/4 teaspoon ground ginger

Sprinkle pork cutlets with red pepper and garlic salt. Place pork in a 4- or 5-quart slow cooker. Halve squash lengthwise; remove and discard seeds. Peel and cut crosswise into 1/2-inch-thick slices; add to slow cooker. Top with sliced oranges, then a combination of cinnamon, cloves, and ginger. Cover and cook on LOW about 4 hours or until pork is tender.

Per serving: Cal 245 · Carb 15 gm · Prot 22 gm · Total fat 11 gm · Sat fat 4 gm · Cal from fat 99 · Chol 59 mg · Sodium 252 mg

PORK WITH SWEET POTATOES, APPLES, AND SAUERKRAUT

*W*hen arranging vegetables in the pot, save the sauerkraut for the top, to provide some flavorful moisture for the ingredients in the bottom.

MAKES 5 SERVINGS

2 medium sweet potatoes

1 medium onion, sliced

2 apples, cored and sliced

1 tablespoon brown sugar

1/4 teaspoon ground cinnamon or nutmeg

1/4 teaspoon salt

1/8 teaspoon ground black pepper

5 boneless pork chops or pork steaks

1 (15- or 16-oz.) can sauerkraut, drained

Peel and cut sweet potatoes into slices about 1/2 inch thick. Arrange over bottom of a 3 1/2-quart slow cooker. Cover with onion, then apples. Sprinkle with brown sugar, cinnamon or nutmeg, salt, and pepper. Top with pork chops, then sauerkraut. Cover and cook on LOW about 5 hours or until chops are tender.

Per serving: Cal 300 · Carb 27 gm · Prot 23 gm · Total fat 11 gm · Sat fat 4 gm · Cal from fat 99 · Chol 59 mg · Sodium 718 mg

COUNTRY-STYLE RIBS WITH GINGER-NECTARINE CHUTNEY

*B*e sure to use large country-style ribs with lots of meat attached to the bones, or substitute lean pork chops or cutlets.

MAKES 6 SERVINGS

1/2 teaspoon curry powder

1/4 teaspoon ground cumin

1/4 teaspoon salt

6 country-style pork ribs

Ginger-Nectarine Chutney

2 nectarines, pitted and chopped

1/4 cup chopped golden raisins

2 tablespoons chopped pecans

1 teaspoon grated gingerroot

2 tablespoons brown sugar

2 teaspoons fresh lemon juice

1/8 teaspoon hot pepper sauce

Combine curry, cumin, and salt in a small bowl. Sprinkle on ribs. Place ribs in a 3 1/2-quart slow cooker. Cover and cook on LOW 4 to 5 hours or until ribs are tender. Prepare chutney while ribs cook: Combine nectarines, raisins, pecans, ginger, sugar, lemon juice, and hot pepper sauce in a small bowl. Spoon chutney over cooked, drained ribs.

Per serving: Cal 277 · Carb 15 gm · Prot 15 gm · Total fat 17 gm · Sat fat 5 gm · Cal from fat 153 · Chol 59 mg · Sodium 140 mg

CANTONESE-STYLE SLOW-COOKED PORK

*T*he results will be just as delicious if you wish to substitute skinned turkey or chicken for the pork.

MAKES ABOUT 4 SERVINGS

3/4 pound boneless lean pork, cut into strips

2 carrots, peeled and coarsely shredded

1 onion, chopped

1 red bell pepper, cut into 1/2-inch squares

2 cups small broccoli flowerets

2 tablespoons soy sauce

1 clove garlic, crushed

2 teaspoons grated gingerroot

1 tablespoon light brown sugar

1/4 teaspoon ground black pepper

Cooked rice

Combine pork, carrots, onion, bell pepper, and broccoli in a 3 1/2-quart slow cooker. In a small bowl, combine soy sauce, garlic, ginger, brown sugar, and pepper. Pour over pork and vegetables. Cover and cook on LOW 6 to 7 hours or until pork is tender. Serve over cooked rice.

Per serving without rice: Cal 175 · Carb 13 gm · Prot 20 gm · Total fat 5 gm · Sat fat 2 gm · Cal from fat 45 · Chol 56 mg · Sodium 582 mg

ALOHA PORK 'N' RICE

*P*eanut butter and chile add flavor keynotes to traditional Hawaiian pork.

MAKES 4 SERVINGS

3/4 pound boneless lean pork

1 red bell pepper, cut into small strips

1/4 cup crunchy-style peanut butter

1 tablespoon honey

1 tablespoon finely chopped candied ginger

1 small jalapeño chile, seeded and minced

2 tablespoons teriyaki sauce

1/2 cup Basmati rice

2 tablespoons coconut, toasted (see Note below)

Cut pork into 1 x 1/4-inch strips. Place pork and bell pepper in a 3 1/2-quart slow cooker. In a small bowl, combine peanut butter, honey, ginger, and jalapeño chile. Stir in teriyaki sauce. Spoon over pork. Cover and cook on LOW 4 or 5 hours or until pork is tender. Stir thoroughly before serving. Meanwhile, cook rice according to package directions. Spoon pork mixture over rice. Sprinkle with toasted coconut.

Per serving: Cal 325 · Carb 28 gm · Prot 24 gm · Total fat 14 gm · Sat fat 4 gm · Cal from fat 126 · Chol 56 mg · Sodium 423 mg

NOTE: Preheat oven to 350F (175C). Spread coconut in a 9-inch pie or cake pan. Toast about 5 minutes or until golden.

VIETNAMESE PORK IN SAVOY CABBAGE

*T*hese miniature bundles of pork-filled cabbage leaves are as appetizing as they look. If you can't find savoy cabbage, use small green cabbage or lettuce leaves.

MAKES 20 SMALL CABBAGE ROLLS

20 leaves Savoy cabbage

1 pound lean ground pork

1/4 cup chopped water chestnuts

1 large clove garlic, minced

3 tablespoons minced green onions, including tops

2 tablespoons minced fresh mint leaves

1 1/2 teaspoons minced gingerroot

1 1/2 teaspoons fresh lemon juice

1/4 teaspoon Chinese hot chili oil

1/4 teaspoon sugar

1/8 teaspoon salt

Sauce

1/3 cup soy sauce

3 tablespoons fresh lemon juice

1 1/2 teaspoons sugar

1 1/2 teaspoons minced gingerroot

1/4 teaspoon Chinese hot chili oil

1 medium clove garlic, minced

1 1/2 teaspoons minced fresh cilantro

1 1/2 teaspoons minced fresh mint leaves

Drop cabbage leaves into boiling water and cook 1 or 2 minutes or until pliable. Immediately plunge into cold water to stop cooking; drain well.

Use a trivet or crumble a large sheet of foil into bottom of slow cooker to keep rolls out of liquid. Cut a "V" from stem end of cabbage leaf; remove tough portion.

In a medium bowl, combine pork, water chestnuts, garlic, green onions, mint, ginger, lemon juice, chili oil, sugar, and salt. Place about 1 1/2 tablespoons pork mixture in center of each cabbage leaf. Roll to enclose mixture. Place on trivet or foil, seam side down, stacking if necessary. Cover and cook on LOW 5 to 6 hours.

Meanwhile, make sauce: Bring all sauce ingredients to a boil in a small saucepan over medium heat, stirring constantly. Reduce heat and simmer 2 to 3 minutes. Remove cabbage rolls to a serving dish. Pour sauce over rolls.

Per cabbage roll: Cal 103 · Carb 5 gm · Prot 6 gm · Total fat 7 gm · Sat fat 1 gm · Cal from fat 63 · Chol 15 mg · Sodium 306 mg

GRACE'S SPECIAL DOLMAS

*T*his popular Middle Eastern dish is an ideal addition to your buffet table. The dolmas (stuffed grape leaves) are delicious served warm or at room tememperature.

MAKES 30 TO 33 DOLMAS

1 large onion, finely chopped

1/2 pound lean ground lamb

2 tablespoons extra-virgin olive oil

1/2 cup long-grain white rice

1 medium tomato, peeled, seeded, and finely chopped

1/4 teaspoon ground allspice

3/4 teaspoon salt

1/2 teaspoon ground black pepper

1/2 cup water

2 tablespoons minced fresh parsley

2 tablespoons minced fresh mint leaves

1 (8-oz.) jar grape leaves in brine

2 cloves garlic, slivered

1 cup fat-free chicken broth or water

6 tablespoons fresh lemon juice

1 medium lemon, cut into wedges (optional)

In a heavy skillet over medium heat, sauté onion and lamb in 1 tablespoon olive oil for 3 minutes, stirring to break up lamb. Add rice and cook, stirring, about 5 minutes. Stir in tomato, allspice, salt, pepper, and water. Cover and simmer 8 to 10 minutes or until the liquid is completely absorbed. Remove from heat. Stir in parsley and mint; set aside to cool.

Rinse and carefully separate grape leaves in a bowl of cold water. Remove stems, if necessary. Cover the bottom of slow cooker with 4 or 5 grape leaves, using any torn ones. Set aside four or five more.

On a work surface, lay remaining grape leaves out flat, rough or vein side up. Place a rounded tablespoon of rice mixture on center of each grape leaf. Fold stem end up over filling, then both sides to middle. Roll up, rather tight, like a small cylinder.

Place dolmas, seam side down, in a 3 1/2-quart slow cooker, layering if necessary. Insert slivers of garlic between rolls. Combine chicken broth or water, remaining 1 tablespoon olive oil, and 3 tablespoons of the lemon juice; pour over rolls. Add a layer of reserved grape leaves. Top with an inverted plate. Cover and cook on LOW 4 to 5 hours or until leaves are tender.

Remove plate and arrange rolls on a serving plate. Drizzle with remaining 3 tablespoons lemon juice and garnish with lemon wedges, if using. Serve warm or at room temperature.

Per dolma: Cal 33 · Carb 3 gm · Prot 2 gm · Total fat 1 gm · Sat fat 0 gm · Cal from fat 9 · Chol 5 mg · Sodium 95 mg

GREEK LAMB, VEGETABLES, AND FETA CHEESE

*P*ackets of tasty morsels are presented on individual dinner plates. Diners slit and pull back the foil to reveal the treasure inside.

MAKES 4 SERVINGS

1 pound lean lamb, cut into bite-size pieces

4 small yellow crookneck squash, cut into 1/4-inch-thick slices

1/4 cup thinly sliced green onions, including tops

1 small red bell pepper, cut into 1-inch cubes

2 ounces feta cheese, diced

1 teaspoon dried oregano leaves

1/2 teaspoon garlic powder

1 teaspoon salt (optional)

1/4 teaspoon ground black pepper

4 teaspoons fresh lemon juice

1/4 cup water

4 lemon wedges

Cut 4 sheets of foil, about 18 x 11 inches each. Place foil, shiny side down, on work surface. Spray an area about the size of a salad plate in center of each piece with nonstick olive oil spray. Top each foil piece with 1/4 of the lamb, then with 1/4 of the squash, then 1/4 of the green onions, bell pepper, and feta cheese. Sprinkle each portion with 1/4 of the oregano leaves, garlic powder, salt, and black pepper. Drizzle each with 1 teaspoon lemon juice. Bring short sides of foil together; fold over twice. Fold sides up twice to seal. Place in a 4-quart slow cooker with folded side up. Pour water around packets. Cover and cook on LOW 6 to 7 hours or until lamb is tender.

To serve, place each sealed packet on a dinner plate. Garnish each with a wedge of lemon.

Per serving: Cal 206 · Carb 6 gm · Prot 26 gm · Total fat 8 gm ·
Sat fat 4 gm · Cal from fat 72 · Chol 84 mg · Sodium 229 mg ½C 3½P

LAMB SHANKS WITH SWEET POTATOES AND DRIED FRUIT

*I*n addition to convenience, a slow cooker also ensures flavorful results.

MAKES ABOUT 6 SERVINGS

2 medium sweet potatoes, peeled and cut crosswise into
   thick slices
1 (8-oz.) package mixed dried fruit
3 or 4 (1- to 1 1/2-lb.) lamb shanks
1/2 cup orange juice
1/2 teaspoon ground cinnamon
1/4 teaspoon ground nutmeg
1 clove garlic, crushed
1/4 teaspoon salt
1/8 teaspoon ground black pepper

Place sweet potatoes on bottom of a 5-quart slow cooker. Top with dried fruit and lamb shanks. In a small bowl, combine orange juice, cinnamon, nutmeg, garlic, salt, and pepper. Pour over lamb. Cover and cook on LOW 8 to 10 hours or until lamb is tender.

Per serving: Cal 285 · Carb 36 gm · Prot 25 gm · Total fat 5 gm · Sat fat 2 gm · Cal from fat 45 · Chol 72 mg · Sodium 181 mg

GARLIC LAMB DIJON

*S*erve these flavor-filled lamb chops with cooked green peas or steamed green beans to round out the meal.

MAKES 4 SERVINGS

1/2 cup Dijon mustard

2 large cloves garlic, minced

1 1/2 tablespoons mustard seeds

1 tablespoon minced fresh rosemary

1/4 teaspoon ground black pepper

4 well-trimmed lean shoulder lamb chops

1/2 teaspoon paprika

Hot cooked rice

Fresh rosemary sprigs for garnish

Combine mustard, garlic, mustard seeds, minced rosemary, and black pepper in a small bowl. Spread mixture (about 1 tablespoon per side) evenly over both sides of lamb chops. Sprinkle top side of each chop with 1/8 teaspoon paprika. Arrange in a 3 1/2-quart slow cooker, overlapping if necessary. Cover and cook on LOW 5 hours or until lamb is tender.

Serve chops with hot cooked rice and the cooking juices. Garnish with rosemary sprigs.

Per serving without rice: Cal 140 · Carb 1 gm · Prot 16 gm · Total fat 8 gm · Sat fat 3 gm · Cal from fat 72 · Chol 52 mg · Sodium 123 mg

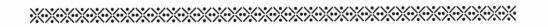

GOOD EATING WITH WRAPS AND SANDWICHES

Your slow cooker is an ideal way to cook a variety of the ingredients that are used for the popular "wraps" or "pita pockets." In these sandwiches the meat or poultry is combined with seasonings and vegetables to make a complete meal. With the slow cooker, you can cook all the ingredients together, then slice or chop the meat or poultry. Keep the mixture warm in the slow cooker until you are ready to stuff the pita pockets or fill the tortillas.

RANGOON CHICKEN WRAPS

*S*easoned with light coconut milk, chutney, gingerroot, and lime peel, this richly flavored wrap includes fragrant jasmine rice.

MAKES 8 WRAPS

1 (4-lb.) whole roasting chicken

2 carrots, peeled and julienned

1 green bell pepper, seeded and sliced

2 tablespoons fruit chutney

1/3 cup crunchy peanut butter

2 tablespoons soy sauce

1 tablespoon grated gingerroot

1/2 teaspoon grated lime peel

1/2 cup unsweetened reduced-fat coconut milk

1/2 cup chicken broth or bouillon

1 cup water

1/2 cup jasmine rice

8 (9-inch) sesame or spinach flour tortillas

8 to 10 snow peas

Remove excess fat from chicken. Remove giblets from chicken and refrigerate for another use. Rinse and drain chicken. Place carrots in a 4- or 5-quart slow cooker. Top with chicken, breast side down, then add bell pepper. Finely chop fruit pieces in chutney; combine in a small bowl with peanut butter, soy sauce, ginger, and lime peel. Stir in coconut milk, then broth. Pour over chicken. Cover and cook on LOW about 5 hours or until chicken is tender.

In a small saucepan, bring water to a boil. Stir in rice. Reduce heat, cover, and cook over low heat about 15 minutes or until rice is tender.

Remove chicken from slow cooker. Remove and discard bones and skin and slice meat.

Fill tortillas with chicken, rice, bell pepper, and carrots. Spoon about 1 1/2 tablespoons cooking juices over each. Cut snow peas into thin strips. Sprinkle on top of filling. Fold ends in and roll up.

Per wrap: Cal 630 · Carb 38 gm · Prot 52 gm · Total fat 30 gm · Sat fat 8 gm · Cal from fat 270 · Chol 113 mg · Sodium 590 mg

HOME-STYLE BARBECUE BEEF WRAPS

A flavorful tri-tip beef roast is a wonderful filling.

MAKES 7 WRAPS

1 (2-lb.) boneless beef loin tri-tip roast

1/4 cup molasses

2 tablespoons prepared mustard

1 tablespoon vinegar

1 teaspoon chili powder

1 tablespoon Worcestershire sauce

1/2 cup ketchup

1 tablespoon minced green onion, including tops

7 (9-inch) chili-flavored or plain flour tortillas

1 (15-oz.) can chili beans, drained, not rinsed, and slightly mashed

1 (11-oz.) can whole-kernel corn, drained

Place beef in a 3 1/2-quart slow cooker. Combine molasses, mustard, vinegar, chili powder, Worcestershire sauce, ketchup, and green onion. Pour half of sauce over beef. Cover and refrigerate remaining sauce. Cover and cook on LOW about 7 hours or until beef is tender.

Preheat oven to 350F (175C). Thinly slice beef across grain. Place about 1/2 cup beef on each tortilla. Top each with about 3 tablespoons beans, 3 tablespoons corn, and 1 tablespoon of the reserved sauce. Fold ends in and roll up. Wrap each in foil. Place in oven about 15 minutes or until heated through.

Per wrap: Cal 528 · Carb 53 gm · Prot 34 gm · Total fat 20 gm · Sat fat 6 gm · Cal from fat 180 · Chol 78 mg · Sodium 458 mg

ALSATIAN PORK WRAPS

*I*f you are a real mashed potato fan, use fresh potatoes.

MAKES 6 WRAPS

1/2 small head cabbage, shredded (about 4 cups)

2 medium apples, peeled, cored, and cut into 8 wedges

1 (3-lb.) sirloin-cut pork roast with bone

2 tablespoons sweet-hot mustard

1/4 teaspoon ground cinnamon

1 teaspoon chili powder

1 tablespoon honey

1/2 teaspoon seasoned salt

1/8 teaspoon ground black pepper

3 (20 x 13-inch) sheets soft Armenian cracker bread

3/4 cup instant mashed potatoes

Hot pepper sauce (optional)

Place cabbage in bottom of a 3 1/2-quart slow cooker; top with apples. Trim and discard any excess fat from pork. Add pork to slow cooker. In a small bowl, combine mustard, cinnamon, chili powder, honey, seasoned salt, and pepper. Spoon over contents of slow cooker. Cover and cook on LOW 7 1/2 to 8 hours or until pork is tender. Remove pork from slow cooker and cut into thin slices. Cut each cracker bread in half. Prepare potatoes according to package directions. Place about 2/3 cup pork on each bread half. Top with about 1/3 cup cabbage mixture and a scant 1/3 cup mashed potatoes, then 2 tablespoons of cooking juices. Fold in sides and roll up. Pass hot sauce, if desired.

Per wrap: Cal 520 · Carb 55 gm · Prot 36 gm · Total fat 17 gm ·
Sat fat 5 gm · Cal from fat 153 · Chol 78 mg · Sodium 548 mg

PESTO- AND TURKEY-STUFFED
PITA POCKETS

*T*his is a half-size version of the popular wraps, featuring pita bread.

MAKES 7 OR 8 SERVINGS

2 uncooked turkey thighs

1 (8-oz.) can sliced water chestnuts, drained

2 cups broccoli flowerets

1 red bell pepper, sliced

1/2 teaspoon salt

1/8 teaspoon ground black pepper

2 teaspoons dry chicken bouillon granules

1 cup lightly packed fresh basil leaves

1/2 cup lightly packed fresh parsley leaves

1 clove garlic, peeled

2 teaspoons vegetable oil

8 ounces (about 1 cup) low-fat or nonfat ricotta cheese

7 or 8 (5- to 6-inch) pita bread rounds, halved crosswise

Remove and discard skin and excess fat from turkey thighs. Rinse turkey and pat dry with paper towels. Place turkey in a 3 1/2-quart slow cooker. Add water chestnuts, broccoli, and bell pepper. Sprinkle with salt, black pepper, and bouillon granules. Cover and cook on LOW for 5 to 6 hours.

In a blender or food processor, combine basil, parsley, garlic, oil, and ricotta cheese. Process until finely chopped.

Remove turkey meat from bones; cut meat into 1-inch strips. Spoon turkey, water chestnuts, broccoli, and green pepper into pita pockets. Top with basil mixture.

Per serving: Cal 233 · Carb 30 gm · Prot 15 gm · Total fat 6 gm · Sat fat 2 gm · Cal from fat 54 · Chol 30 mg · Sodium 556 mg

TACO-SEASONED TURKEY PITAS

*T*his hearty and healthy dish is great for lunch or for impressing friends at a Sunday night supper.

MAKES ABOUT 8 SERVINGS

3/4 pound lean ground turkey

3 green onions, including tops, sliced

1 (1-oz.) package dry taco spices and seasonings

1 large bunch spinach, washed, stemmed, and cut into
   1/4-inch slices

2 carrots, peeled and shredded

8 pita bread rounds

Combine turkey, green onions, taco mix, spinach, and carrots in a 3 1/2-quart slow cooker. Stir to mix well. Cover and cook on LOW about 4 hours or until onions are tender.

Stir turkey mixture and let stand while heating pita rounds or for at least 5 minutes.

Preheat oven to 350F (175C). Halve pita rounds crosswise and place on a baking sheet. Heat pita rounds until warmed, about 10 minutes. Fill pita rounds with turkey mixture and serve.

Per serving: Cal 179 · Carb 23 gm · Prot 11 gm · Total fat 4 gm · Sat fat 1 gm · Cal from fat 36 · Chol 34 mg · Sodium 318 mg

TERIYAKI BEEF PITAS

Serve with beans or rice for a more complete meal.

MAKES 5 OR 6 SERVINGS

3/4 pound lean beef round steak

1/2 cup teriyaki sauce

2 stalks celery, sliced

1/2 teaspoon dried thyme

1 medium onion, sliced

1 clove garlic, chopped

1/8 teaspoon ground black pepper

2 tablespoons cornstarch

2 tablespoons cold water

5 to 6 pita pocket rounds

Shredded lettuce

Cut round steak into about 2 x 1/4-inch strips. Place in a 3 1/2-quart slow cooker. Top with teriyaki sauce, celery, thyme, onion, garlic, and pepper. Cover and cook on LOW 6 to 7 hours or until steak is tender. Turn control to HIGH. In a small bowl, dissolve cornstarch in cold water. Stir into contents of slow cooker. Cover and cook, stirring occasionally, 15 to 20 minutes or until thickened.

Slice about 1 inch off 1 side of each pita round. Spoon steak mixture into pita rounds; top with shredded lettuce.

Per serving: Cal 288 · Carb 30 gm · Prot 19 gm · Total fat 9 gm · Sat fat 2 gm · Cal from fat 81 · Chol 41 mg · Sodium 1367 mg

PELE'S HOT CHICKEN SANDWICH

*T*his colorful and tasty topping for an open-face hot sandwich borrows flavors from the South Pacific.

MAKES 4 OR 5 SERVINGS

1 pound boneless, skinless chicken breasts, cut into 2 x 1/2-
 inch strips

1 red bell pepper, cut into julienne strips

1 zucchini, cut into julienne strips

6 mushrooms, sliced

3/4 cup pineapple juice

2 tablespoons teriyaki sauce

1 tablespoon honey

1/2 teaspoon salt

1/8 to 1/4 teaspoon dried red pepper flakes

2 tablespoons cornstarch

2 tablespoons cold water

4 to 5 sesame bagels

1 small jicama, peeled and coarsely shredded

Combine chicken, bell pepper, zucchini, mushrooms, juice, teriyaki sauce, honey, salt, and pepper flakes in a 3 1/2-quart slow cooker. Cover and cook on LOW about 4 hours or until chicken is tender.

Turn control to HIGH. In a small bowl, dissolve cornstarch in cold water. Stir into contents of slow cooker. Cover and cook 15 to 20 minutes or until thickened.

Meanwhile, preheat broiler. Split bagels and place, cut sides up, on a baking sheet. Toast under broiler until lightly browned, about 5 minutes. Serve chicken mixture on bagels. Top with jicama.

Per serving: Cal 373 · Carb 51 gm · Prot 34 gm · Total fat 3 gm · Sat fat 1 gm · Cal from fat 27 · Chol 39 mg · Sodium 856 mg

BARBECUED BEEF 'N' BEAN BURGERS

*S*o good to eat but so messy to pick up—it's best to serve these sandwiches with a knife and fork.

MAKES 5 OR 6 SERVINGS

1 (15-oz.) can small white or red beans, drained

3 green onions, including tops, chopped

2 stalks celery, finely chopped

1/2 pound extra-lean ground beef, crumbled into small
   pieces

1 (8-oz.) can tomato sauce

1/4 teaspoon liquid smoke

1 tablespoon honey

1/4 teaspoon grated lemon peel

5 or 6 hamburger buns

Spoon drained beans into a 3 1/2-quart slow cooker. Add green onions, celery, ground beef, tomato sauce, liquid smoke, honey, and lemon peel. Stir until thoroughly combined. Cover and cook on LOW about 4 hours or until vegetables are tender.

Preheat broiler. Split buns and place, cut sides up, on a baking sheet. Toast under broiler until lightly browned, about 5 minutes. Serve bean mixture on toasted buns.

Per serving: Cal 356 · Carb 48 gm · Prot 19 gm · Total fat 10 gm · Sat fat 7 gm · Cal from fat 90 · Chol 31 mg · Sodium 558 mg

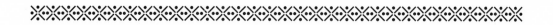

SLOW-AND-EASY
BEANS AND GRAINS

*A*ll of us are aware that dried beans cooked the conventional way take a long time to prepare. After much experimenting with dried beans in slow cookers, we prefer the following method for most basic recipes: Combine dried beans with water and seasonings (including sauces, tomatoes, spices, onions, and meat). Cover and cook on HIGH for the number of hours indicated in the individual recipe. Usually, this is 8 to 10 hours.

A more traditional method that also works well but takes longer is: Soak 1 pound dried beans in 6 cups water overnight in a slow cooker. Cover and cook on HIGH 2 or 3 hours or until tender. Drain, saving liquid. Return beans to slow cooker. Stir in desired seasonings and 1 cup reserved liquid from beans. Cover and cook on LOW 10 to 12 hours.

CANNELLINI AND SALMON SALAD TOSS

*F*or eye appeal, save a few of the large fennel leaves to use as a garnish.

MAKES 6 OR 7 SERVINGS

1 pound dried cannellini beans, sorted and rinsed

7 cups water

1 1/2 teaspoons salt

1 small fennel bulb, finely chopped or sliced and leaves
   reserved for garnish

1 small red onion, chopped

2 carrots, peeled and thinly sliced

2 tablespoons chopped fresh dill

1/3 cup vegetable oil

2 tablespoons fresh lemon juice

1/8 teaspoon ground black pepper

1/2 pound fresh salmon fillets or thin salmon steaks

Combine beans, water, and 1 teaspoon salt in a 3 1/2-quart slow cooker. Cover and cook on HIGH 9 to 10 hours or until beans are tender.

Dip out beans with slotted spoon, draining off liquid. Refrigerate beans until chilled.

In a large bowl, combine chilled beans, fennel, onion, carrots, dill, oil, lemon juice, remaining 1/2 teaspoon salt, and pepper.

Preheat broiler. Rinse salmon and place on a broiler rack. Broil salmon until it just begins to flake when pierced with a fork, about 10 minutes. Break salmon into chunks and remove any bones. Sprinkle salmon over fennel mixture. Garnish with fennel leaves.

Per serving: Cal 450 · Carb 50 gm · Prot 23 gm · Total fat 18 gm · Sat fat 2 gm · Cal from fat 162 · Chol 21 mg · Sodium 412 mg

SPICY PINTOS ON TORTILLAS

*T*hese are designed for those who enjoy bean dishes with a chile accent.

MAKES 12 TORTILLAS

1 pound dried pinto or kidney beans, sorted and rinsed

1 jalapeño chile, seeded and chopped

1 mild green chile, seeded and chopped

1 medium red onion, chopped

1 clove garlic, crushed

1/4 cup chopped fresh parsley

2 tablespoons chopped fresh cilantro

1/2 teaspoon salt

1/4 teaspoon ground black pepper

1 teaspoon chili powder

4 cups beef broth

1 cup water

1 tablespoon vegetable oil

12 medium flour tortillas

Shredded Cheddar cheese (optional)

Combine beans, chiles, onion, garlic, parsley, cilantro, salt, pepper, chili powder, broth, and water in a 3 1/2-quart slow cooker. Cover and cook on HIGH about 6 hours or until beans are tender.

Heat oil in a large skillet over medium heat. Adding 1 or 2 tortillas at a time, heat until lightly browned; turn and brown other side. Repeat until all are browned. Dip out beans with a slotted spoon, draining off liquid. Use beans as a topping for tortillas. Sprinkle with cheese, if desired.

Per tortilla: Cal 254 · Carb 42 gm · Prot 12 gm · Total fat 5 gm · Sat fat 0.5 gm · Cal from fat 45 · Chol 0 mg · Sodium 363 mg

BARBECUED PINTO BEANS

*T*hese beans are the perfect accompaniment for your favorite grilled steaks or burgers.

MAKES 6 TO 8 SERVINGS

1 pound dried pinto beans, sorted and rinsed

3 cups water

1 onion, chopped

1 green bell pepper, chopped

1 jalapeño chile, seeded and chopped

1 (18-oz.) bottle barbecue sauce

1/4 cup molasses

1/4 teaspoon salt

Combine all ingredients in a 3 1/2-quart slow cooker. Cover and cook on HIGH 8 to 9 hours or until beans are tender.

Per serving: Cal 374 · Carb 66 gm · Prot 17 gm · Total fat 5 gm · Sat fat 0 gm · Cal from fat 45 · Chol 0 mg · Sodium 812 mg

TASTE-OF-ITALY BEANS 'N' SAUSAGE

*T*his is a slow-cooker version of a popular traditional main dish from the hill towns of Italy.

MAKES ABOUT 8 SERVINGS

1 pound dried cannellini beans or lima beans, sorted and
    rinsed

4 cups water

1 clove garlic, crushed

1 (14 1/2-oz.) can diced tomatoes with Italian seasoning

1 tablespoon chopped fresh sage leaves

1/2 to 3/4 pound sweet Italian turkey sausage, crumbled

1/2 teaspoon salt

1/4 teaspoon ground black pepper

Combine all ingredients in a 3 1/2-quart slow cooker. Cover and cook on HIGH 9 to 10 hours or until beans are tender.

Per serving: Cal 265 · Carb 39 gm · Prot 17 gm · Total fat 5 gm · Sat fat 0 gm · Cal from fat 45 · Chol 15 mg · Sodium 502 mg

BARBECUED LIMAS AND BEEF

*C*hoose high or low cooking, depending on which method fits into your schedule.

MAKES 5 OR 6 SERVINGS

1 pound dried small lima beans, sorted and rinsed

1/2 pound beef stew meat, cut into 1/4-inch cubes

1 small onion, chopped

2 stalks celery, chopped

1 carrot, coarsely shredded

1/4 teaspoon salt

1/8 teaspoon ground black pepper

1/2 cup barbecue sauce

1 (6-oz.) can tomato paste

1 tablespoon prepared mustard

1 tablespoon honey

4 cups water

Combine beans, beef, onion, celery, carrot, salt, and pepper in a 3 1/2-quart slow cooker. Stir in barbecue sauce, tomato paste, mustard, honey, and water. Cover and cook on LOW 10 hours or cook on HIGH 5 1/2 to 6 hours, stirring once, or until beans and beef are tender.

Per serving: Cal 494 · Carb 71 gm · Prot 30 gm · Total fat 11 gm · Sat fat 2 gm · Cal from fat 99 · Chol 27 mg · Sodium 437 mg

BAKED BEANS WITH CANADIAN BACON

*I*t is important to thoroughly stir the mixture at least once to ensure even cooking for all the beans.

MAKES 6 TO 8 SERVINGS

1 pound dried small white beans, sorted and rinsed

4 cups water

1/3 cup molasses

1/4 cup packed light brown sugar

1 medium onion, chopped

1 tablespoon prepared mustard

1/2 teaspoon salt

2 ounces sliced Canadian bacon, cut into strips

Thoroughly combine beans, water, molasses, brown sugar, onion, mustard, and salt in a 3 1/2-quart slow cooker. Place bacon strips on top. Cover and cook on HIGH about 5 hours. Stir mixture; cover and cook on HIGH 1 to 2 additional hours or until beans are tender.

Per serving: Cal 365 · Carb 66 gm · Prot 17 gm · Total fat 4 gm · Sat fat 0 gm · Cal from fat 36 · Chol 3 mg · Sodium 340 mg

PICANTE BEEF 'N' BEANS

*T*ake this dish to your next potluck dinner and impress your friends.

MAKES 6 TO 8 SERVINGS

1 pound dried red kidney beans, sorted and rinsed

1 large red onion, thinly sliced

2 medium tomatoes, chopped

2 tablespoons chopped fresh cilantro

1/2 pound lean beef round steak, cut into strips about
   1/4-inch thick

1 (8-oz.) jar picante sauce

2 (10 1/2-oz.) cans condensed beef bouillon

Combine kidney beans, onion, tomatoes, and cilantro in a 3 1/2-quart slow cooker. Top with beef, then picante sauce and beef bouillon. Cover and cook on LOW 8 to 8 1/2 hours or until beans and beef are tender.

Per serving: Cal 498 · Carb 66 gm · Prot 31 gm · Total fat 13 gm · Sat fat 3 gm · Cal from fat 117 · Chol 38 mg · Sodium 821 mg

SPICED GARBANZO BEANS

*T*his vegetarian delight features an exciting combination of spices to liven up garbanzo beans (also called chickpeas).

MAKES 6 OR 7 SERVINGS

2 (15-oz.) cans garbanzo beans

1 medium onion, chopped

1 inch piece fresh gingerroot, peeled and finely chopped

3 cloves garlic, minced

1 (14 1/2-oz.) can diced tomatoes in juice

1 teaspoon ground black pepper

1 teaspoon ground cloves

1/2 teaspoon ground cardamom

1/2 teaspoon ground coriander

1 teaspoon ground cumin

2 bay leaves

1 (1-inch) piece stick cinnamon

3 dried red chiles

1/2 teaspoon salt

Chopped cilantro

Drain garbanzo beans; reserve 3/4 cup liquid. Combine drained garbanzo beans, onion, ginger, and garlic in a 3 1/2-quart slow cooker. Add 3/4 cup reserved liquid and diced tomatoes with juice. Stir in pepper, cloves, cardamom, coriander, cumin, bay leaves, cinnamon, dried chiles, and salt. Cover and cook on LOW 8 to 9 hours. Remove and discard bay leaves, cinnamon stick, and chiles. Sprinkle with chopped cilantro.

Per serving: Cal 163 · Carb 29 gm · Prot 7 gm · Total fat 3 gm · Sat fat 0 gm · Cal from fat 37 · Chol 0 mg · Sodium 854 mg

EASY THREE-BEAN MEDLEY

*E*qually delicious whether served as a snack with chips or spread on tortillas as a favorite lunch, this dish cooks quickly because you start with canned beans.

MAKES ABOUT 6 CUPS

1 (15-oz.) can red beans, drained and rinsed

1 (15-oz.) can black beans, drained and rinsed

1 (8 3/4-oz.) can red kidney beans, drained and rinsed

1 large tomato, chopped

1 clove garlic, crushed

2 tablespoons chopped fresh cilantro

1 teaspoon chili powder

1 small cucumber

1 cup picante sauce

Tortillas or corn chips

Shredded reduced-fat Cheddar cheese or low-fat sour
    cream (optional)

Combine beans, tomato, garlic, cilantro, and chili powder in a 3 1/2-quart slow cooker. Peel cucumber and halve lengthwise. Scoop out and discard seeds. Dice cucumber and stir into beans. Stir in picante sauce. Cover and cook on LOW about 4 hours. Spoon beans onto tortillas or dip corn chips into warm mixture. Sprinkle with cheese or sour cream, if desired.

Per cup without tortillas: Cal 187 · Carb 36 gm · Prot 11 gm ·
Total fat 1 gm · Sat fat 0 gm · Cal from fat 9 · Chol 0 mg ·
Sodium 963 mg

CURRIED LENTILS AND VEGETABLES

*L*ightly cooking the spices together before they are added to the other ingredients is the secret to a very special flavor combination. Be very careful not to burn them.

MAKES 5 OR 6 SERVINGS

1 1/2 cups baby carrots

1 cup thinly sliced celery

1 small onion, minced

2 medium yams, peeled and diced

1 cup dried lentils, sorted and rinsed

2 teaspoons vegetable oil

1 clove garlic, minced

1 tablespoon curry powder

1 teaspoon ground cumin

1/2 teaspoon salt

1/4 teaspoon ground white pepper

1 teaspoon minced gingerroot

1 (14 1/2-oz.) can fat-free chicken broth

1 tablespoon minced lemon peel

1/2 cup frozen green peas

1/2 cup nonfat plain yogurt

2 tablespoons minced green onion, including top

Combine carrots, celery, onion, yams, and lentils in a 3 1/2-quart slow cooker; set aside.

Heat oil in a small skillet over medium heat. Add garlic, curry powder, cumin, salt, pepper, and ginger. Cook, stirring, 1 minute. Stir in chicken broth and lemon peel. Pour over vegetables in slow cooker. Cover and cook on LOW 6 to 7 hours or until vegetables are tender.

Turn control to HIGH. Place frozen peas in a strainer. Run hot water over them to thaw. Add peas to contents of slow cooker. Cover and cook on HIGH 15 minutes. Top each serving with a dab of yogurt and a sprinkle of green onion.

Per serving: Cal 182 · Carb 38 gm · Prot 10 gm · Total fat 3 gm · Sat fat 0.5 gm · Cal from fat 27 · Chol 1 mg · Sodium 491 mg

VEGETARIAN SOYBEANS

A garden of summer vegetables enhances this meatless dish.

MAKES 6 TO 8 SERVINGS

1 pound dried soybeans, sorted and rinsed

1 cup water

4 cups vegetable juice

2 zucchini, shredded

2 tomatoes, chopped

1 yellow bell pepper, chopped

1 jalapeño chile, seeded and minced

1 onion, chopped

2 tablespoons chopped fresh cilantro

2 teaspoons chili powder

1 clove garlic, crushed

Combine all ingredients in a 3 1/2-quart slow cooker. Cover and cook on HIGH 8 to 9 hours, stirring once after 7 hours if possible, or until beans are tender.

Per serving: Cal 382 · Carb 36 gm · Prot 29 gm · Total fat 15 gm · Sat fat 2 gm · Cal from fat 135 · Chol 0 mg · Sodium 146 mg

BARLEY AND BEEF STEW

*T*his chunky stew is hearty enough to serve as a main dish.

MAKES ABOUT 6 SERVINGS

1/2 pound beef stew meat or round steak, cut into 1/2-
   inch cubes
3/4 cup pearl barley
4 carrots, peeled and sliced
2 stalks celery with leaves, chopped
1 large onion, chopped
2 turnips, peeled and cut into 1/2-inch cubes
1 teaspoon dried thyme leaves
1/2 teaspoon salt
1/4 teaspoon ground black pepper
5 cups beef broth

Combine beef, barley, carrots, celery, onion, turnips, thyme, salt, and pepper in a 3 1/2-quart slow cooker. Pour in broth. Cover and cook on LOW 9 to 11 hours or until beef and barley are tender. Spoon into soup bowls.

Per serving: Cal 223 · Carb 30 gm · Prot 13 gm · Total fat 6 gm · Sat fat 2 gm · Cal from fat 54 · Chol 23 mg · Sodium 886 mg

STUFFED GRAPE LEAVES

*F*or a strictly vegetarian dish, substitute vegetable broth for the chicken broth.

MAKES 22 TO 25 GRAPE ROLLS

1/2 cup uncooked long-grain white rice

1 cup fat-free chicken broth

2 tablespoons chopped fresh parsley

1 small onion, finely chopped

1/4 teaspoon salt

1/8 teaspoon ground black pepper

1/8 teaspoon ground allspice

1/4 teaspoon grated lemon peel

1/4 cup dried currants

2 tablespoons pine nuts, toasted (see Note opposite)

1 (8-oz.) jar grape leaves (40 to 45 leaves)

In a medium saucepan, combine rice, broth, parsley, onion, salt, pepper, allspice, and lemon peel. Cover and simmer gently over low heat 15 minutes or until rice is tender. Stir in currants and pine nuts; set aside.

Rinse and carefully separate grape leaves in a bowl of cold water. Remove stems, if necessary. Set aside 22 to 25 of the most perfect ones. Place a metal rack in bottom of a 3 1/2-quart slow cooker. Top with the imperfect leaves.

On a work surface, lay perfect leaves out flat, rough or vein side up. Spoon about 1 1/2 to 2 tablespoons stuffing near stem end of each leaf. Fold stem end up over filling, then both sides to middle. Roll up, rather tight, like a small cylinder. Stack rolls very close together on bed of leaves in slow cooker. Top with an inverted heavy plate to hold rolls in place. Add enough hot water to cover rolls. Cover and cook on LOW 6 to 7 hours or until leaves are tender. Drain and serve warm or at room temperature.

Per grape roll: Cal 26 · Carb 5 gm · Prot 1 gm · Total fat 0.5 gm · Sat fat 0 gm · Cal from fat 5 · Chol 0 mg · Sodium 74 mg

NOTE: Preheat oven to 350F (175C). Spread nuts in a 9-inch pie or cake pan. Toast 5 to 8 minutes or until golden. Or toast nuts in a dry skillet over low heat 3 or 4 minutes.

WILD RICE
WITH PORTOBELLO MUSHROOMS

*P*ortobello mushrooms add a meatlike flavor and texture.

MAKES 5 OR 6 SERVINGS

3/4 cup wild rice, rinsed and drained

1/2 cup long-grain brown rice

1/2 pound portobello mushrooms, stems removed

1 medium onion, diced

2 cups diced celery

1/2 pound boneless lean pork, cut into 1/2-inch cubes

1 (10 3/4-oz.) can reduced-fat cream of mushroom soup

1/4 teaspoon ground sage

1/4 teaspoon ground black pepper

2 cups hot chicken broth or bouillon

1/4 cup soy sauce

1/4 cup minced fresh parsley

1/4 cup slivered almonds (optional), toasted (see Note,
  page 165)

Combine rices in a 3 1/2-quart slow cooker. Wipe mushrooms with a damp cloth. Cut into 3/8-inch-thick slices; add to slow cooker. Stir in onion, celery, pork, soup, sage, and pepper. Stir in broth and soy sauce. Cover and cook on LOW 6 to 7 hours or until all the liquid is absorbed and rices are tender. Stir before serving. Garnish each serving with minced fresh parsley and toasted almonds, if desired.

Per serving: Cal 314 · Carb 44 gm · Prot 19 gm · Total fat 8 gm ·
Sat fat 2 gm · Cal from fat 72 · Chol 31 mg · Sodium 1576 mg

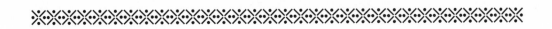

FROM THE GARDEN
TO THE SLOW COOKER

With an increased emphasis on the nutritional value of fresh vegetables in our diets, we have become interested in using them in a variety of ways. Our slow-cooker vegetable dishes range from appetizers to main dishes and many of them offer a combination of two or more compatible vegetables.

For an impressive, aromatic vegetable combination, you will enjoy Sorrento Potato and Cheese Packets. Potatoes, pearl onions, and cherry tomatoes are packed in foil with herbs and cheese, then cooked on a trivet in the slow cooker.

Shells of many fresh vegetables make attractive, appetizing, and flavorful containers for main dishes. We especially enjoy red or green bell peppers stuffed with a well-seasoned combination of smoked turkey sausage and corn (see page 177).

SICILIAN SALSA

*F*or a change, try this salsa with your favorite pasta.

MAKES 6 TO 8 SERVINGS

2 medium eggplants, peeled and diced

1/2 cup chopped onion

1/2 cup diced celery

3 large cloves garlic, minced

1 (6-oz.) can tomato paste

3 tablespoons red wine vinegar

1 tablespoon olive oil

1/2 teaspoon dried oregano leaves, crushed

1/2 teaspoon dried basil leaves, crushed

1/2 teaspoon ground black pepper

1/4 cup capers, drained

1/4 cup small pimiento-stuffed olives, thinly sliced

3 tablespoons minced fresh parsley

1 1/2 tablespoons pine nuts, toasted (see Note, page 165)

1 loaf French or Italian bread, thinly sliced

Combine eggplant, onion, celery, garlic, tomato paste, vinegar, olive oil, oregano, basil, and pepper in a 3 1/2-quart slow cooker. Cover and cook on LOW 6 to 8 hours or until eggplants are tender. Stir in capers, olives, parsley, and pine nuts. Serve at room temperature or chilled. To serve, spoon on sliced French or Italian bread.

Per serving: Cal 288 · Carb 46 gm · Prot 9 gm · Total fat 9 gm · Sat fat 1 gm · Cal from fat 288 · Chol 0 mg · Sodium 767 mg

CURRIED CAULIFLOWER APPETIZER

Choose a firm, compact, creamy white head of cauliflower for an attractive presentation.

MAKES 12 TO 16 SERVINGS

1 large (about 2 1/2-lb.) head cauliflower

1/2 cup water

1 tablespoon fresh lemon juice

1/2 cup light mayonnaise

1/2 cup nonfat plain yogurt

1/4 teaspoon ground ginger

1/4 teaspoon salt

1/4 teaspoon ground white pepper

1 teaspoon curry powder

Fresh sprigs of parsley, for garnish

Paprika, for garnish (optional)

Wheat crackers (optional)

Remove and discard outer leaves of cauliflower. Cut out core, about 1 1/2 inches deep. Place cauliflower, stem side down, in a 3 1/2-quart slow cooker. Combine water and lemon juice. Pour over cauliflower. Cover and cook on LOW 4 to 6 hours or until very tender. Meanwhile, in a small bowl, mix mayonnaise, yogurt, ginger, salt, pepper, and curry powder. Cover and refrigerate at least 1 hour for flavors to blend. Arrange cauliflower on a serving plate. Spread mayonnaise mixture evenly over cooked cauliflower. Surround with sprigs of fresh parsley. Dust the top lightly with paprika and serve with crackers, if desired.

Per serving: Cal 46 · Carb 7 gm · Prot 3 gm · Total fat 2 gm · Sat fat 0 gm · Cal from fat 18 · Chol 2 mg · Sodium 106 mg

EGGPLANT & SQUASH VEGGIE DIP

*T*his dip is somewhat chunky; if you prefer a smoother texture, slightly mash cooked mixture with a fork.

MAKES 3 1/2 TO 4 CUPS

1 medium eggplant, peeled and cut into 1/2-inch cubes

1 medium butternut squash, peeled, seeded, and cut into
   1/2-inch cubes

1 onion, chopped

1 mild green chile, seeded and diced

1 clove garlic, crushed

1 tablespoon vegetable oil

1 tablespoon red wine vinegar

1 teaspoon honey

1/2 teaspoon salt

2 tablespoons chopped fresh cilantro

1 teaspoon chopped fresh basil

Pita bread, cut into wedges, or corn chips

Combine eggplant, butternut squash, onion, chile, garlic, oil, vinegar, honey, and salt in a 3 1/2-quart slow cooker. Cover and cook on LOW about 7 hours or until vegetables are tender.

Stir in cilantro and basil. Transfer to a serving bowl, cover, and refrigerate until chilled. Serve as a dip with pita bread or corn chips.

Per 1/4 cup: Cal 29 · Carb 5 gm · Prot 0 gm · Total fat 1 gm · Sat fat 0 gm · Cal from fat 9 · Chol 0 mg · Sodium 77 mg

SUMMER VEGETABLE MEDLEY

A great hot-weather, fresh vegetable combination that won't heat up your kitchen—serve it as a side dish. (*See photo on cover.*)

MAKES 4 OR 5 SERVINGS

3 medium zucchini, coarsely chopped

1 ear of corn, kernels cut off the cob

1 leek, cleaned and thinly sliced

1 jalapeño chile, seeded and minced

1 clove garlic, minced

3 medium tomatoes, peeled and coarsely chopped

1 tablespoon margarine or butter

1/2 teaspoon seasoned salt

1/4 teaspoon ground black pepper

Combine zucchini, corn, leek, jalapeño chile, and garlic in a 3 1/2-quart slow cooker. Top with tomatoes. Dot with margarine or butter, then sprinkle with seasoned salt and pepper. Cover and cook on LOW about 5 hours. Spoon into a serving dish.

Per serving: Cal 104 · Carb 18 gm · Prot 3 gm · Total fat 4 gm · Sat fat 0 gm · Cal from fat 36 · Chol 0 mg · Sodium 311 mg

✗ SORRENTO POTATO AND CHEESE PACKETS

*T*he potatoes absorb the rich flavors of the Mediterranean, releasing a mouth-watering aroma when the packet is opened.

MAKES 6 SERVINGS

6 medium red potatoes, cut into eighths

18 pearl onions, trimmed and peeled

18 cherry tomatoes

6 cloves garlic, thinly sliced

4 to 6 ounces goat or feta cheese, crumbled

About 2 tablespoons olive oil

1 tablespoon finely chopped fresh rosemary

1 1/2 teaspoons dried oregano leaves, crushed

1/2 teaspoon salt

1/4 teaspoon ground black pepper

Cut 6 (15 x 12-inch) sheets of foil. For each serving, place 1 potato, 3 onions, and 3 cherry tomatoes in center of each foil sheet. Sprinkle each serving with 1 garlic clove, then 1/6 of the cheese. Drizzle each with about 1/2 teaspoon olive oil, and then sprinkle with equal amounts of rosemary, oregano, salt, and pepper. Bring short ends of foil together; fold over twice to seal. Insert trivet in bottom of a 3 1/2-quart slow cooker; pour in 1/4 cup water. Arrange foil packets on trivet. Cover pot and cook on LOW about 8 hours or until vegetables are tender. To serve, place 1 packet on each plate.

Per serving: Cal 262 · Carb 40 gm · Prot 7 gm · Total fat 9 gm · Sat fat 3 gm · Cal from fat 81 · Chol 17 mg · Sodium 406 mg

GINGERED CARROTS WITH DIJON MUSTARD AND BROWN SUGAR

*F*or an easy way to fix carrots for a family get-together, cook and serve in the slow cooker.

MAKES 10 TO 12 SERVINGS

12 to 14 medium carrots, cut into sticks about 2 x 1/2
   inches
1 tablespoon margarine or butter, at room temperature
1/3 cup Dijon mustard
1/2 cup packed light brown sugar
1 teaspoon grated gingerroot

Place carrots in a 3 1/2-quart slow cooker. In a small bowl, combine margarine or butter, mustard, brown sugar, and ginger; stir into carrots. Cover and cook on HIGH for 2 to 3 hours or until carrots are tender.

Per serving: Cal 89 · Carb 19 gm · Prot 1 gm · Total fat 1 gm · Sat fat 0 gm · Cal from fat 9 · Chol 0 mg · Sodium 67 mg

SPICY EGGPLANT WITH PINE NUTS

*A*n exciting yet easy way to add interest to a vegetable dish.

MAKES 6 OR 7 SERVINGS

1 large eggplant

1 medium onion, thinly sliced

1 jalapeño chile, seeded and chopped

1 clove garlic, minced

1 medium tomato, chopped

1/4 teaspoon salt

1/8 teaspoon ground black pepper

1/4 teaspoon ground cumin

2 teaspoons vegetable or olive oil

3 tablespoons pine nuts

Cut eggplant crosswise into 3/4-inch slices; place in a 3 1/2-quart slow cooker. Top with onion, jalapeño chile, garlic, tomato, salt, pepper, and cumin. Cover and cook on LOW about 5 hours or until eggplant is tender.

While eggplant cooks, heat oil in a small skillet over medium heat. Add pine nuts and sauté, stirring, until golden, about 3 minutes. Transfer eggplant to a serving dish and sprinkle with pine nuts.

Per serving: Cal 61 · Carb 6 gm · Prot 1 gm · Total fat 4 gm · Sat fat 0 gm · Cal from fat 36 · Chol 0 mg · Sodium 93 mg

RAGOUT OF RED CABBAGE
WITH PORT

*S*erve as an accompaniment to roast pork, ham, or duck.

MAKES ABOUT 10 SERVINGS

1 medium head (about 2 lbs.) red cabbage

1 large red onion, chopped

1 medium apple, cored and chopped

Peel of 1/2 large orange, orange part only, cut into fine
   slivers

2 tablespoons sugar

1 teaspoon salt

1/2 teaspoon ground black pepper

1/2 cup port or other sweet red wine

1 tablespoon cornstarch

1/4 cup red wine vinegar

1/2 to 1 teaspoon caraway seeds, crushed (optional)

Finely shred cabbage. Combine cabbage, onion, apple, orange peel, sugar, salt, pepper, and wine in a 3 1/2-quart slow cooker. Cover and cook on LOW 7 to 8 hours or until vegetables are tender. Turn control to HIGH. In a small bowl, dissolve cornstarch in vinegar. Add to cabbage mixture and stir. Cover and cook on HIGH 15 to 20 minutes or until slightly thickened. Add caraway, if desired.

Per serving: Cal 63 · Carb 12 gm · Prot 1 gm · Total fat 0 gm · Sat fat 0 gm · Cal from fat 0 · Chol 0 mg · Sodium 224 mg

SWEET-AND-SOUR SQUASH

*S*erve as a Moroccan-inspired vegetable dish with traditional meats or as an accompaniment to couscous.

MAKES 4 OR 5 SERVINGS

3/4-lb. uncooked unpeeled banana squash

2 large leaves uncooked kale

3 oz. Canadian bacon, chopped

3/4 cup sweet-and-sour sauce

Remove and discard peel from squash; cut into 1/2-inch pieces. Place squash on bottom of a 3 1/2-quart slow cooker. Trim kale and cut crosswise into 1/2-inch strips; add to squash. Sprinkle the vegetables with bacon. Spoon sweet-and-sour sauce over all. Cover and cook on LOW 4 to 4 1/2 hours or until squash is tender.

Per serving: Cal 118 · Carb 22 gm · Prot 4 gm · Total fat 2 gm · Sat fat 0 gm · Cal from fat 18 · Chol 8 mg · Sodium 358 mg

CORN- AND TURKEY-STUFFED BELL PEPPERS

*T*his colorful main dish is loaded with important nutrients.

MAKES 6 SERVINGS

1/2 pound smoked turkey sausage, finely chopped

1 medium onion, finely chopped

1 (11-oz.) can whole-kernel corn, drained

2 slices toasted bread, crusts removed and cubed

2 tablespoons chopped fresh parsley

1/2 teaspoon salt

1/8 teaspoon ground black pepper

1 teaspoon chopped fresh thyme or 1/4 teaspoon dried

2 medium tomatoes, seeded, peeled, and chopped

3 large red or green bell peppers, cut in half lengthwise
   and seeded

In a large bowl, combine turkey sausage, onion, corn, bread, parsley, salt, black pepper, thyme, and tomatoes. Spoon into pepper halves. Arrange on bottom of a 3 1/2-quart slow cooker, stacking if necessary. Cover and cook on LOW about 5 hours or until peppers are tender.

Per serving: Cal 150 · Carb 21 gm · Prot 9 gm · Total fat 4 gm · Sat fat 1 gm · Cal from fat 36 · Chol 20 mg · Sodium 665 mg

PORK- AND CHUTNEY-STUFFED ONIONS

*A*n appetizing way to use leftover roast pork—serve as a light main dish or as a side dish.

MAKES 5 SERVINGS

5 medium (about 8 oz. each) onions

2 cups chopped cooked boneless pork roast or cutlets (about 8 oz.)

1/4 cup soft bread crumbs

1 tablespoon chopped fresh parsley

1/8 teaspoon Italian seasoning

2 tablespoons fruit chutney, fruit finely chopped

1/4 teaspoon salt

1/8 teaspoon ground black pepper

1 to 2 tablespoons coconut, toasted (see Note, page 127), or chopped cashews

Cut off about a 1/2-inch slice from top of each onion. Peel onions and scoop out centers, leaving about 1/2-inch-thick sides and bottoms. In a medium bowl, combine pork, bread crumbs, parsley, Italian seasoning, chutney, salt, and pepper. Spoon into onion shells. Place onions on bottom of a 4- to 5-quart slow cooker. Cover and cook on LOW 7 to 8 hours or until onions are done. Sprinkle with coconut or cashews.

Per serving: Cal 168 · Carb 23 gm · Prot 12 gm · Total fat 3 gm · Sat fat 1 gm · Cal from fat 27 · Chol 30 mg · Sodium 200 mg

CLASSIC TOMATO-VEGETABLE PASTA SAUCE

*S*tir in 1 tablespoon fresh basil when making the sauce, then sprinkle an extra teaspoon on top of the finished dish for extra eye appeal and flavor.

MAKES 4 OR 5 SERVINGS

1 (28-oz.) can tomato puree

2 stalks celery, chopped

2 medium leeks, chopped and rinsed

1 cup sliced fresh mushrooms

1 clove garlic, crushed

1/4 cup dry red wine

1 tablespoon chopped fresh basil

1/4 teaspoon salt

1/8 teaspoon ground black pepper

12 ounces spaghetti or noodles

1 teaspoon finely chopped fresh basil

Combine tomato puree, celery, leeks, mushrooms, garlic, wine, 1 tablespoon chopped basil, salt, and pepper in a 3 1/2-quart slow cooker. Cover and cook on LOW 6 to 7 hours or until vegetables are tender.

Cook pasta according to package directions. Drain and transfer to a serving bowl. Spoon sauce over pasta. Sprinkle sauce with finely chopped basil.

Per serving: Cal 453 · Carb 94 gm · Prot 16 gm · Total fat 2 gm · Sat fat 0 gm · Cal from fat 18 · Chol 0 mg · Sodium 963 mg

STEAMED BROCCOLI-CORN PUDDING

*F*resh corn and broccoli are combined in this vegetable casserole.

MAKES 5 OR 6 SERVINGS

2 ears of corn

2 eggs, slightly beaten

1 cup evaporated skim milk

1 small bunch (about 1/2 lb.) fresh broccoli, finely
   chopped

1/4 cup yellow cornmeal

1/2 teaspoon chili powder

1/8 teaspoon ground black pepper

1/4 teaspoon salt

2 tablespoons grated Parmesan cheese

Grease bottom and sides of a 6-cup baking dish or metal bowl that fits into a slow cooker; set aside.

Cut corn kernels off cobs. In a medium bowl, combine corn, eggs, milk, broccoli, cornmeal, chili powder, pepper, and salt. Pour into prepared dish. Sprinkle with Parmesan cheese. Cover with foil, crimping edges to seal.

Pour 2 cups hot water into a 4- to 5-quart slow cooker and add a metal rack. Set casserole on rack in slow cooker. Cover and cook on HIGH 2 1/2 to 3 hours or until a knife inserted in mixture comes out clean. Serve warm from baking dish.

Per serving: Cal 151 · Carb 21 gm · Prot 10 gm · Total fat 4 gm ·
Sat fat 1 gm · Cal from fat 36 · Chol 89 mg · Sodium 262 mg

BAKED ONIONS AND APPLES WITH CINNAMON

*T*his fills your kitchen with a wonderful aroma while it is cooking!

MAKES 6 TO 8 SERVINGS

2 large onions, cut in half from top to bottom, then
  crosswise in thin slices

1/2 teaspoon salt

1/4 teaspoon ground black pepper

4 large baking apples, cored and thinly sliced

2 tablespoons sugar

1 teaspoon ground cinnamon

2 tablespoons margarine or butter

2 tablespoons chopped pecans (optional)

Arrange half of the onion slices in a 3 1/2-quart slow cooker; sprinkle with half of the salt and pepper. Top with half of the apples; sprinkle with half the sugar and cinnamon. Repeat layers with remaining ingredients. Dot top with margarine or butter. Cover and cook on LOW 8 hours or until onions and apples are tender. Top with chopped pecans, if desired.

Per serving: Cal 137 · Carb 26 gm · Prot 1 gm · Total fat 4 gm · Sat fat 1 gm · Cal from fat 36 · Chol 0 mg · Sodium 224 mg

POTATO AND TURNIP SLICES WITH MUSTARD AND HORSERADISH

*T*his appealing combination will entice almost anyone to enjoy vegetables.

MAKES 6 OR 7 SERVINGS

1 (5-oz.) can evaporated skim milk

1 tablespoon sweet-hot mustard

1 tablespoon prepared horseradish

1/2 teaspoon salt

1/8 teaspoon ground black pepper

1/8 teaspoon ground nutmeg

5 medium potatoes, peeled and thinly sliced

3 medium turnips, peeled and thinly sliced

1 tablespoon chopped fresh chives

In a small bowl, combine milk, mustard, horseradish, salt, pepper, and nutmeg. Place half of the potatoes into a 3 1/2-quart slow cooker; top with half the turnips. Spoon half of the milk mixture over all. Repeat with remaining potatoes, turnips, and milk mixture. Sprinkle with chopped chives. Cover and cook on LOW about 5 hours or until vegetables are tender.

Per serving: Cal 128 · Carb 28 gm · Prot 4 gm · Total fat 0 gm · Sat fat 0 gm · Cal from fat 0 · Chol 1 mg · Sodium 271 mg

GOLDEN DELICIOUS APPLES AND YAM SCALLOP

*T*he cinnamon- and nutmeg-accented apples and yams are a perfect fall dish to accompany a ham or a pork roast.

MAKES 6 TO 8 SERVINGS

- 5 or 6 medium yams, peeled and cut into 1/2-inch-thick slices
- 3 medium Golden Delicious apples, cored and cut into 1/2-inch-thick slices
- 3 tablespoons fresh lemon juice
- 3/4 cup lightly packed light brown sugar
- 1 tablespoon all-purpose flour
- 1 teaspoon ground cinnamon
- 1/4 teaspoon ground nutmeg
- 1/4 teaspoon salt
- 1/4 teaspoon ground white pepper
- 1/4 cup chopped pecans
- 1 tablespoon margarine or butter (optional)

In a large bowl, combine yams, apples, and lemon juice; toss to coat. In a small bowl, combine brown sugar, flour, cinnamon, nutmeg, salt, pepper, and pecans. Place half of the yam mixture in a 4- to 5-quart slow cooker; top with half of the brown sugar mixture. Repeat with remaining yam mixture and brown sugar mixture. Dot top with margarine or butter, if desired. Cover and cook on LOW 7 to 8 hours or until yams and apples are tender.

Per serving: Cal 275 · Carb 62 gm · Prot 2 gm · Total fat 3 gm · Sat fat 0 gm · Cal from fat 27 · Chol 0 mg · Sodium 107 mg

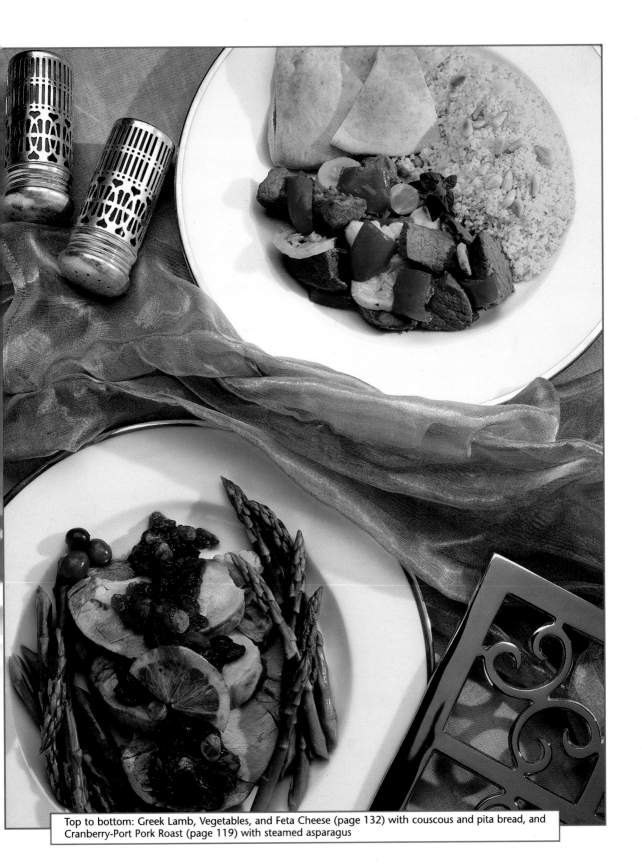

Top to bottom: Greek Lamb, Vegetables, and Feta Cheese (page 132) with couscous and pita bread, and Cranberry-Port Pork Roast (page 119) with steamed asparagus

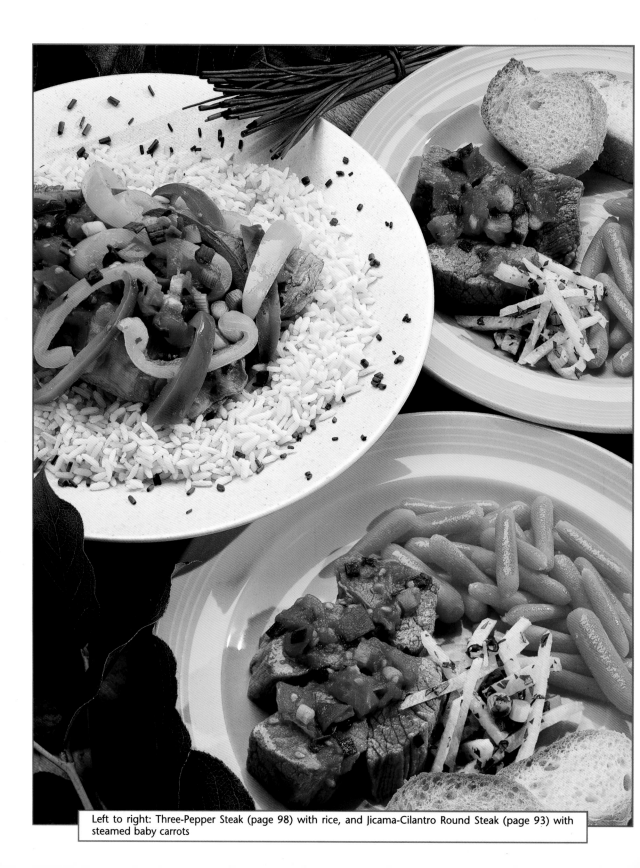

Left to right: Three-Pepper Steak (page 98) with rice, and Jicama-Cilantro Round Steak (page 93) with steamed baby carrots

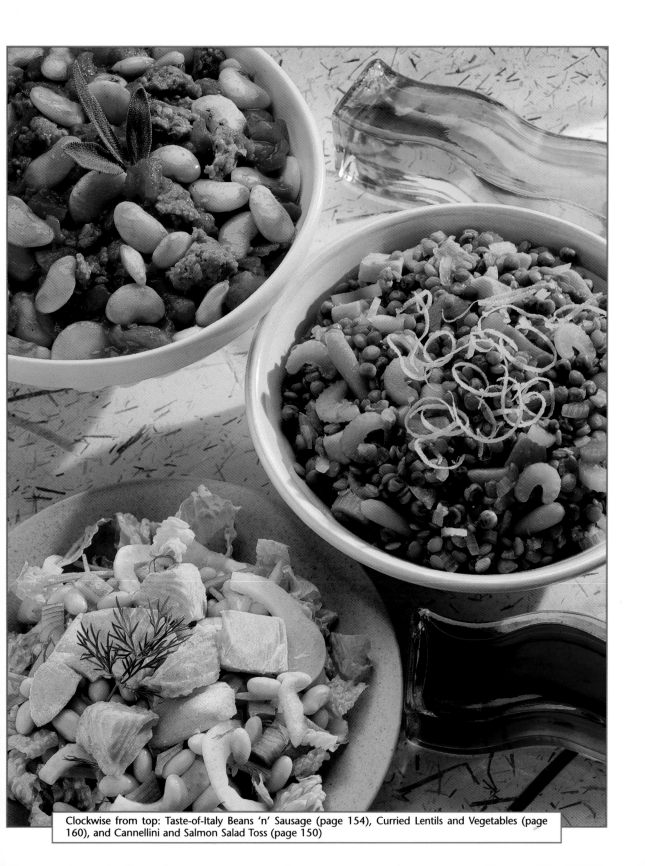

Clockwise from top: Taste-of-Italy Beans 'n' Sausage (page 154), Curried Lentils and Vegetables (page 160), and Cannellini and Salmon Salad Toss (page 150)

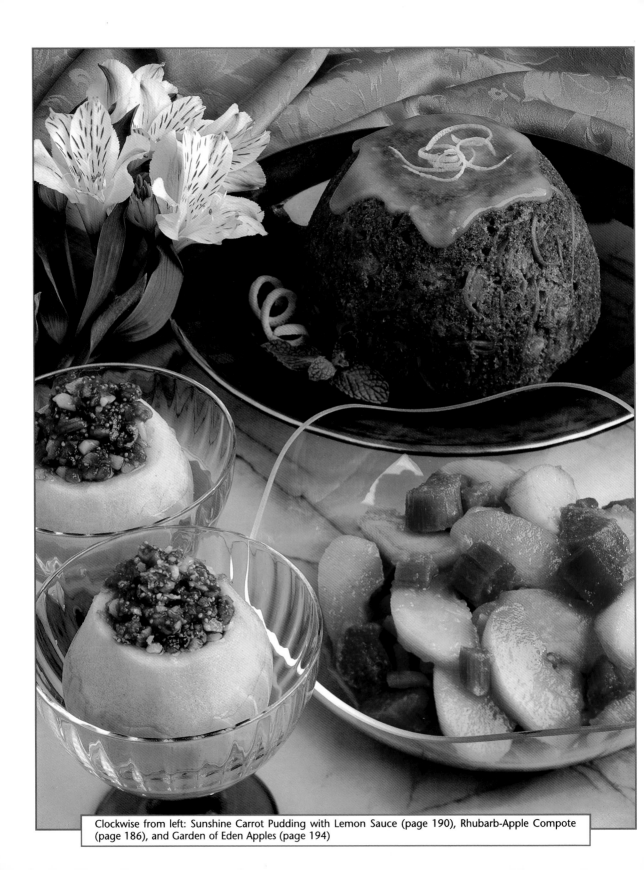

Clockwise from left: Sunshine Carrot Pudding with Lemon Sauce (page 190), Rhubarb-Apple Compote (page 186), and Garden of Eden Apples (page 194)

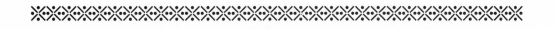

YEAR-ROUND DESSERTS
AND ACCOMPANIMENTS

Your slow cooker may not be the most practical appliance for baking a traditional pie or cake, but it is ideal for a wide variety of other desserts. Cooks who enjoy steamed puddings are enthusiastic about the results from slow cooking. At Thanksgiving imagine surprising your guests with Pumpkin-Date Pudding with Rum Sauce as a break from the traditional pie. Or try Sunshine Carrot Pudding with Lemon Sauce with a base of whole-wheat and white flours that is enhanced with a mellow spice mixture and pineapple-raisin accents. For the holiday season, you will be proud to serve Steamed Cranberry Pudding with Orange Blossom Sauce. Cooking the dessert in the slow cooker frees up space in your oven for other dishes.

Family-favorite recipes of baked apples prepared in the slow cooker are very popular. Garden of Eden Apples with figs and almonds, as well as Slow-Cooker Baked Cranberry Apples, are especially appropriate for the fall and winter seasons.

RHUBARB-APPLE COMPOTE

Choose firm, bright red stalks of rhubarb for this fruit-filled treat.

MAKES 5 OR 6 SERVINGS

1 pound fresh rhubarb, cut into 1-inch pieces

4 large cooking apples, peeled, cored, and cut into thin
   wedges

1/2 cup sugar

2 teaspoons minced candied ginger

1 teaspoon grated orange peel

1/4 cup apple juice

Ground nutmeg

Combine rhubarb, apples, sugar, candied ginger, orange peel, and apple juice in a 3 1/2- or 4-quart slow cooker. Cover and cook on LOW about 5 hours or until rhubarb and apples are soft.

Spoon into dessert dishes. Sprinkle with nutmeg.

Per serving: Cal 178 · Carb 46 gm · Prot 1 gm · Total fat 1 gm · Sat fat 0 gm · Cal from fat 9 · Chol 0 mg · Sodium 5 mg

CHUNKY BLACK CHERRY APPLESAUCE

*T*he combination of flavors in this sauce are so interesting that it can serve as an accompaniment to pork chops or roast as well as a satisfying dessert.

MAKES ABOUT 6 1/2 CUPS

8 large apples
1 (16-oz.) package frozen unsweetened pitted dark sweet
    cherries
1/2 cup sugar
1/4 teaspoon ground nutmeg
1/2 teaspoon ground cinnamon
1/4 teaspoon almond extract

Peel and core apples. Cut apples into 1/2-inch pieces. Combine apples, frozen cherries, sugar, nutmeg, cinnamon, and almond extract in a 3 1/2-quart slow cooker. Cover and cook on LOW about 10 hours or until fruit is very soft. Transfer to a bowl and refrigerate until cold.

Per 1/2 cup: Cal 121 · Carb 31 gm · Prot 1 gm · Total fat 0 gm · Sat fat 0 gm · Cal from fat 0 · Chol 0 mg · Sodium 1 mg

STEAMED PUMPKIN-DATE PUDDING WITH RUM SAUCE

*I*f you don't have pumpkin pie spice, use 1/2 teaspoon cinnamon and 1/4 teaspoon *each* allspice, cloves, and ginger.

MAKES 10 SERVINGS

1 1/2 cups all-purpose flour

1/2 cup packed light brown sugar

1 teaspoon baking powder

1/2 teaspoon baking soda

1 1/2 teaspoons pumpkin pie spice

1/4 teaspoon salt

1 cup canned pumpkin

2 tablespoons lemon yogurt

1 teaspoon vanilla extract

1/2 cup chopped dates

Rum Sauce

1/3 cup sugar

4 teaspoons cornstarch

1/4 teaspoon ground nutmeg

Pinch of salt

2/3 cup water

1/4 cup light rum

1 teaspoon margarine or butter

Spray a 6-cup metal mold with vegetable cooking spray; set aside. Place a trivet in bottom of a 4- to 5-quart or larger slow cooker.

In a medium bowl, stir together flour, brown sugar, baking powder, baking soda, pumpkin pie spice, and salt. Add pumpkin, yogurt, and vanilla and mix until combined. Stir in dates. Spoon batter into prepared mold; cover with a lid or foil secured with string. Place mold on trivet in slow cooker. Cover and cook on HIGH 3 hours or until a wooden pick inserted in center comes out clean.

Meanwhile, prepare Rum Sauce: In a small saucepan, combine sugar, cornstarch, nutmeg, and salt. Gradually stir in water and rum. Cook and stir over low heat until mixture is thickened, about 3 minutes. Remove from heat; stir in margarine or butter. Makes 1 1/8 cups.

Remove mold from slow cooker and remove string and foil. Cool pudding on a wire rack 10 minutes. Loosen edges and turn out pudding onto a serving plate. Slice and serve warm or at room temperature with Rum Sauce.

Per serving: Cal 167 · Carb 35 gm · Prot 3 gm · Total fat 1 gm · Sat fat 0 gm · Cal from fat 9 · Chol 0 mg · Sodium 190 mg

SUNSHINE CARROT PUDDING
WITH LEMON SAUCE

*T*his pudding can be eaten immediately, but the flavor improves if it is allowed to rest 8 hours before serving.

MAKES 8 TO 10 SERVINGS

1 cup whole-wheat flour

1/2 cup all-purpose flour

1/2 cup packed dark brown sugar

1/4 cup granulated sugar

1 teaspoon baking powder

1 teaspoon baking soda

1 teaspoon ground cinnamon

1/2 teaspoon ground nutmeg

1/8 teaspoon ground cloves

1/2 teaspoon salt

2 tablespoons diced candied ginger

2 cups lightly packed shredded carrots

1 (8-oz.) can crushed pineapple in juice

1 teaspoon vanilla extract

1/2 cup golden raisins

Lemon Sauce

1/2 cup sugar

1 1/2 tablespoons cornstarch

3 to 4 tablespoons fresh lemon juice

1 cup water

1 to 2 drops yellow food coloring (optional)

1 teaspoon margarine or butter

Grease and flour a 5- to 6-cup metal mold; set aside. Place a trivet in bottom of a 4- to 5-quart or larger slow cooker.

In a medium bowl, stir together whole-wheat and all-purpose flours, brown and granulated sugars, baking powder, baking soda, cinnamon, nutmeg, cloves, and salt. Add ginger, carrots, pineapple with juice, and vanilla and mix until combined. Batter will be thick. Transfer batter to prepared mold; cover mold with a lid or foil secured with string. Place on trivet in slow cooker. Pour about 1 cup hot water around mold. Cover and cook on HIGH 3 hours or until a wooden pick inserted in center comes out clean.

Remove pudding mold from slow cooker. Remove string and foil. Cool pudding on a wire rack 15 to 20 minutes.

Meanwhile, prepare Lemon Sauce: In a small saucepan, combine sugar and cornstarch. Stir in lemon juice and water. Cook over medium heat, stirring constantly, until mixture comes to a boil and thickens. Remove from heat; stir in food coloring, if using, and butter. Serve warm. Makes about 1 1/3 cups.

Loosen edges and turn out pudding onto a serving plate. Slice and serve warm or at room temperature with warm Lemon Sauce.

Per serving: Cal 198 · Carb 46 gm · Prot 4 gm · Total fat 1 gm · Sat fat 0 gm · Cal from fat 9 · Chol 0 mg · Sodium 298 mg

STEAMED CRANBERRY PUDDING WITH ORANGE BLOSSOM SAUCE

*U*se fresh or frozen cranberries. Freeze fresh cranberries when they are in season for dishes such as this.

MAKES 8 TO 10 SERVINGS

1 1/3 cups all-purpose flour

1 teaspoon baking soda

1/2 teaspoon salt

1/2 teaspoon ground allspice

1/4 teaspoon ground nutmeg

2 cups coarsely chopped fresh cranberries

1/2 cup honey

1/3 cup hot water

Orange Blossom Sauce

2 tablespoons liquid egg substitute

2 tablespoons sugar

1/3 cup frozen orange juice concentrate, thawed

1/3 cup water

1 teaspoon margarine or butter

Grease and flour a 1-quart metal mold; set aside.

In a large bowl, stir together flour, baking soda, salt, allspice, and nutmeg. Add cranberries, honey, and hot water and mix until combined. Spoon into prepared mold. Cover with a lid or foil secured with string. Place mold in a 4-quart or larger slow cooker. Pour 1 cup hot water around mold in slow cooker. Cover and cook on HIGH 3 hours or until a wooden pick inserted in center comes out clean.

Remove pudding mold from slow cooker. Remove string and foil. Cool on a wire rack 15 minutes.

Meanwhile, prepare Orange Blossom Sauce: In a medium saucepan, whisk together egg substitute, sugar, orange juice concentrate, and water. Cook over medium-low heat, stirring constantly, until sauce is thick and creamy, about 5 minutes. Remove from heat, stir in margarine or butter. Serve hot. Makes about 1 cup.

When pudding has cooled, loosen edges and turn out onto a serving plate. Slice pudding and serve warm or at room temperature. Top each serving with hot Orange Blossom Sauce.

Per serving: Cal 185 · Carb 42 gm · Prot 3 gm · Total fat 1 gm · Sat fat 0 gm · Cal from fat 9 · Chol 0 mg · Sodium 250 mg

GARDEN OF EDEN APPLES

*B*efore starting to make this dish, be sure that the apples will fit into your slow cooker; four large apples will not work in smaller pots.

MAKES 4 SERVINGS

3/4 cup chopped dried figs

2 tablespoons chopped blanched almonds

1/3 cup boiling water

1/2 cup honey

1 teaspoon margarine or butter

4 medium to large baking apples

Almond Cream

1/2 cup nonfat sour cream

4 teaspoons powdered sugar

1/4 teaspoon almond extract

In a small bowl, combine figs and almonds; set aside. In another bowl, stir together boiling water, honey, and margarine or butter.

Starting at blossom end, peel apples about 1/3 of the way down; remove most of core and seeds, leaving a small amount of core at bottom. Spoon about 2 tablespoons fig and almond mixture into each apple. Place in a 4-quart or larger slow cooker. Pour honey mixture over apples. Cover and cook on LOW 3 to 4 hours or until apples are tender. Baste apples with cooking juices.

Meanwhile prepare Almond Cream: In a small bowl, mix together all ingredients. Refrigerate at least 1 hour for flavors to mingle. Makes 1/2 cup.

To serve, spoon a little of the honey syrup just off center on each dessert plate. Spoon about 2 tablespoons of the Almond Cream next to it; place an apple on top in center. Repeat on 3 more dessert plates.

Per serving: Cal 377 · Carb 87 gm · Prot 3 gm · Total fat 4 gm · Sat fat 0.5 gm · Cal from fat 36 · Chol 4 mg · Sodium 59 mg

SLOW-COOKER
BAKED CRANBERRY APPLES

*B*e sure to check if all the apples will fit into your slow cooker before peeling them.

MAKES 5 SERVINGS

5 medium baking apples

1/3 cup fresh or frozen cranberries, chopped

1/4 cup packed light brown sugar

1/4 teaspoon ground cinnamon

1/8 teaspoon ground nutmeg

2 tablespoons chopped walnuts

Whipped or sour cream (optional)

Peel each apple about a fourth of the way down; remove core and seeds. In a small bowl, combine cranberries, sugar, cinnamon, nutmeg, and walnuts. Spoon cranberry mixture into center of each apple. Place in a 4-quart or larger slow cooker. Cover and cook on LOW 4 to 5 hours or until apples are tender.

Serve warm or at room temperature. Top with whipped or sour cream, if desired.

Per serving: Cal 132 · Carb 33 gm · Prot 0 gm · Total fat 1 gm · Sat fat 0 gm · Cal from fat 9 · Chol 0 mg · Sodium 4 mg

DRIED CHERRY AND APPLE SNACK

*D*ried tart cherries and oatmeal topping turn ordinary cooking apples into an extraordinary dessert.

MAKES 4 TO 6 SERVINGS

1/2 cup dried pitted tart cherries

1/2 cup apple juice

3 large tart green apples, peeled, cored, and sliced

1/4 cup all-purpose flour

1/2 cup sugar

1/2 teaspoon ground cinnamon

1/2 cup old-fashioned rolled oats

2 tablespoons light brown sugar

2 tablespoons margarine or butter, at room temperature

Place a metal rack in a 4- to 5-quart or larger slow cooker. Grease a 5- or 6-cup mold or baking dish; set aside. In a medium bowl, combine cherries and apple juice; let stand about 1 hour or until reconstituted. Stir in apples.

In a small bowl, combine flour, sugar, and cinnamon. Add flour mixture to cherry mixture and stir until combined. Spoon into greased mold or baking dish.

With a pastry blender, combine oats, brown sugar, and margarine or butter until crumbly. Spoon on top of apple mixture in mold. Cover with foil. Place on rack in slow cooker. Cover and cook on HIGH 4 to 5 hours. Remove mold from slow cooker. Remove foil and let stand 5 minutes. Cut into slices or squares.

Per serving: Cal 389 · Carb 73 gm · Prot 5 gm · Total fat 10 gm · Sat fat 2 gm · Cal from fat 90 · Chol 0 mg · Sodium 104 mg

POACHED APPLES 'N' CRANBERRIES

A delicious way to satisfy one of your daily fruit requirements.

MAKES 6 OR 7 SERVINGS

1 1/2 cups dry red wine

1 cup reduced-calorie cranberry juice

1/3 cup honey

1/4 teaspoon Angostura aromatic bitters

5 cups peeled, thick slices cooking apples

3/4 cup dried cranberries

5 whole allspice

5 whole cloves

1 (3-inch) piece cinnamon stick

Orange Cream

3/4 cup nonfat sour cream

1 1/2 teaspoons grated orange peel

1 1/2 teaspoons sugar

Combine red wine, cranberry juice, honey, and bitters in a 3 1/2-quart slow cooker. Stir until honey is dissolved. Add apples and cranberries; stir to mix. Tie allspice, cloves, and cinnamon in a small piece of cheesecloth or place in a metal spice ball. Bury spices among apples and cranberries. Cover and cook on LOW 5 hours or until apples are tender. Let cool. Meanwhile, make Orange Cream: Combine sour cream, orange rind and sugar in a small bowl. Cover and chill at least 1 hour. Spoon over fruit and cooking juice.

Per serving: Cal 220 · Carb 49 gm · Prot 1 gm · Total fat 0 gm · Sat fat 0 gm · Cal from fat 0 · Chol 4 mg · Sodium 46 mg

PEAR STREUSEL

No need to heat up the kitchen for this lovely and luscious dessert.

MAKES ABOUT 4 SERVINGS

1/3 cup crunchy nutlike cereal nuggets

3 tablespoons all-purpose flour

3 tablespoons light brown sugar

2 tablespoons soft reduced-fat margarine

1 teaspoon grated lemon peel

1/2 teaspoon ground ginger

4 Bartlett pears, peeled, cored, and cut into 1/2-inch slices

3 tablespoons fresh lemon juice

1/4 cup granulated sugar

In a small bowl, combine cereal, flour, brown sugar, margarine, lemon peel, and ginger. Mix with a fork until mixture is crumbly; set aside.

In a 1-quart casserole dish that fits into a 4- or 5-quart slow cooker, combine pears, lemon juice, and granulated sugar. Sprinkle crumb mixture evenly over top. Place casserole in slow cooker. Cover and cook on HIGH 2 hours or until pears are fork tender. Serve warm.

Per serving: Cal 264 · Carb 60 gm · Prot 2 gm · Total fat 4 gm · Sat fat 0.5 gm · Cal from fat 36 · Chol 0 mg · Sodium 134 mg

ALMOND BREAD PUDDING WITH BRANDIED CHERRY SAUCE

*T*he sauce adds flavor and color to this dessert.

MAKES 6 TO 8 SERVINGS

3 cups 1/2-inch French bread cubes

2 1/4 cups low-fat milk

2 eggs

1/2 cup sugar

1/2 teaspoon vanilla extract

1/2 teaspoon almond extract

3 tablespoons sliced almonds, toasted (see Note, page 165)

Brandied Cherry Sauce

1 (20-oz.) can light cherry pie filling

2 1/2 tablespoons brandy

1/4 teaspoon almond extract

Place bread cubes in a 1 1/2 quart casserole that fits into a 4- or 5-quart cooker. In a medium bowl, whisk together milk, eggs, sugar, vanilla, and almond extract. Pour over bread; cover dish with foil and place in slow cooker. Pour 1/2 cup boiling water around casserole. Cover and cook on HIGH 2 hours. Meanwhile, make sauce: Combine all ingredients. Cover and chill at least 1 hour. Makes about 2 cups. Sprinkle pudding with almonds and serve warm or cold with sauce.

Per serving: Cal 220 · Carb 30 gm · Prot 7 gm · Total fat 6 gm · Sat fat 2 gm · Cal from fat 54 · Chol 78 mg · Sodium 160 mg

BRANDIED FRUIT COMPOTE

*T*his is a colorful and glistening medley of flavorful fruits; serve as a wholesome dessert or accompaniment to pork or chicken dishes.

MAKES 12 TO 14 SERVINGS

2 (8-oz.) packages dried mixed fruit

1 cup diced dried pineapple

2/3 cup dried cranberries

1/2 cup golden raisins

1 medium orange

1/2 cup honey

2 cups hot water

3/4 teaspoon ground allspice

1/2 cup brandy

Frozen yogurt or ice cream (optional)

Combine mixed fruit, pineapple, cranberries, and raisins in a 3 1/2-quart slow cooker. Remove a thin layer of orange part of peel from orange; cut into very thin strips. Squeeze juice from orange. Add peel, juice, honey, water, and allspice to slow cooker, stirring until honey is dissolved.

Cover and cook on LOW 5 to 6 hours or until fruit is plump and tender. Stir in brandy; cool. Serve in a compote or over frozen yogurt or ice cream.

Per serving: Cal 185 · Carb 43 gm · Prot 1 gm · Total fat 0 gm · Sat fat 0 gm · Cal from fat 0 · Chol 0 mg · Sodium 20 mg

POLYNESIAN PINEAPPLE-MANGO RELISH

*T*his exotic South Seas combo is guaranteed to perk up your next tropical dinner party. Serve it with poultry or pork.

MAKES ABOUT 4 CUPS

1 small fresh pineapple

1 mango

3/4 cup sugar

2 tablespoons chopped gingerroot

1/2 cup golden raisins

1 jalapeño chile, seeded and chopped

1 onion, coarsely chopped

1 small red or green bell pepper, diced

1 clove garlic, finely chopped

1/4 cup white vinegar

1/8 teaspoon ground turmeric

Peel, core, and dice pineapple. Peel, pit, and dice mango. Combine pineapple and mango in a 3 1/2-quart slow cooker. Stir in sugar, ginger, raisins, jalapeño chile, onion, bell pepper, garlic, vinegar, and turmeric. Cover and cook on LOW about 5 hours or until onion is tender.

Per 1/4 cup: Cal 74 · Carb 19 gm · Prot 0 gm · Total fat 0 gm · Sat fat 0 gm · Cal from fat 0 · Chol 0 mg · Sodium 1 mg

AUTUMN SURPRISE RELISH

*P*acked with the flavor of fruit and spices, this is an interesting accompaniment to baked ham or pork roast.

MAKES ABOUT 3 CUPS

1 cooking apple, peeled, cored, and diced

1 acorn squash, seeded, peeled, and diced

1 orange, peeled, seeded, and diced

1/2 cup dried currants

1/4 teaspoon ground cinnamon

2 tablespoons chopped candied ginger

1/4 cup white vinegar

1/2 cup packed light brown sugar

1/8 teaspoon ground red pepper

Combine apple, squash, orange, and currants in a 3 1/2-quart slow cooker. Stir in cinnamon, ginger, vinegar, brown sugar, and red pepper. Cover and cook on LOW about 8 hours. Turn control to HIGH and cook, uncovered, 2 hours.

Per 1/4 cup: Cal 78 · Carb 20 gm · Prot 1 gm · Total fat 0 gm · Sat fat 0 gm · Cal from fat 0 · Chol 0 mg · Sodium 4 mg

METRIC CONVERSION CHARTS

COMPARISON TO METRIC MEASURE

When You Know	Symbol	Multiply By	To Find	Symbol
teaspoons	tsp.	5.0	milliliters	ml
tablespoons	tbsp.	15.0	milliliters	ml
fluid ounces	fl. oz.	30.0	milliliters	ml
cups	c	0.24	liters	l
pints	pt.	0.47	liters	l
quarts	qt.	0.95	liters	l
ounces	oz.	28.0	grams	g
pounds	lb.	0.45	kilograms	kg
Fahrenheit	F	5/9 (after subtracting 32)	Celsius	C

FAHRENHEIT TO CELSIUS

F	C
200–205	95
220–225	105
245–250	120
275	135
300–305	150
325–330	165
345–350	175
370–375	190
400–405	205
425–430	220
445–450	230
470–475	245
500	260

LIQUID MEASURE TO MILLILITERS

1/4	teaspoon	=	1.25	milliliters
1/2	teaspoon	=	2.5	milliliters
3/4	teaspoon	=	3.75	milliliters
1	teaspoon	=	5.0	milliliters
1-1/4	teaspoons	=	6.25	milliliters
1-1/2	teaspoons	=	7.5	milliliters
1-3/4	teaspoons	=	8.75	milliliters
2	teaspoons	=	10.0	milliliters
1	tablespoon	=	15.0	milliliters
2	tablespoons	=	30.0	milliliters

LIQUID MEASURE TO LITERS

1/4	cup	=	0.06 liters
1/2	cup	=	0.12 liters
3/4	cup	=	0.18 liters
1	cup	=	0.24 liters
1-1/4	cups	=	0.3 liters
1-1/2	cups	=	0.36 liters
2	cups	=	0.48 liters
2-1/2	cups	=	0.6 liters
3	cups	=	0.72 liters
3-1/2	cups	=	0.84 liters
4	cups	=	0.96 liters
4-1/2	cups	=	1.08 liters
5	cups	=	1.2 liters
5-1/2	cups	=	1.32 liters

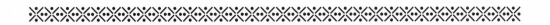

INDEX

Almonds
  Almond Bread Pudding with Brandied Cherry Sauce, 200
  Garden of Eden Apples, 194–195
  Aloha Pork 'n' Rice, 127
  Alsatian Pork Wraps, 141
Angostura aromatic bitters
  Poached Apples 'n' Cranberries, 198
Appetizers
  Curried Cauliflower Appetizer, 169
  Eggplant & Squash Veggie Dip, 170
Apple cider
  Pork and Apple Hot-Pot, 120
Apple juice
  Dried Cherry and Apple Snack, 197
  Turkey, Yam, and Apple Stew, 77
  Rhubarb-Apple Compote, 186
Apples
  Alsatian Pork Wraps, 141
  Autumn Surprise Relish, 203
  Baked Onions and Apples with Cinnamon, 181
  Chicken with Cabbage and Apples, 49
  Chunky Black Cherry Applesauce, 187
  Dried Cherry and Apple Snack, 197
  Garden of Eden Apples, 194–195
  Gold 'n' Green Squash Soup, 12
  Golden Delicious Apples and Yam Scallop, 183
  Poached Apples 'n' Cranberries, 198
  Pork with Sweet Potatoes, Apples, and Sauerkraut, 124
  Pork and Apple Hot-Pot, 120
  Ragout of Red Cabbage with Port, 175
  Rhubarb-Apple Compote, 186

  Slow-Cooker Baked Cranberry Apples, 196
  Turkey, Yam, and Apple Stew, 77
Applesauce
  Chunky Black Cherry Applesauce, 187
Around the World with Chicken, 35–65
Asparagus Cube Steak Roll-Ups, 107
Autumn Surprise Relish, 203
Avocados
  Fresh Salsa, 16
  Pot Roast with Avocado-Chile Topping, 100

Bagels
  Pele's Hot Chicken Sandwich, 146–147
Baked Beans with Canadian Bacon, 156
Baked Onions and Apples with Cinnamon, 181
Barbecue sauce
  Barbecued Limas and Beef, 155
  Barbecued Pinto Beans, 153
Barbecued Beef 'n' Bean Burgers, 148
Barbecued Brisket 'n' Noodles, 99
Barbecued Limas and Beef, 155
Barbecued Pinto Beans, 153
Barley
  Barley and Beef Stew, 163
Basil
  Classic Tomato-Vegetable Pasta Sauce, 179
  Pesto- and Turkey-Stuffed Pita Pockets, 142–143
  Pork Chops with Minted Herb Relish, 122
  Pot Roast with Basil, Sun-Dried Tomatoes, and Pine Nuts, 102

Bean sprouts
  Roasted Chicken Stuffed with Water Chestnuts and Bean Sprouts, 40
Beans
  Baked Beans with Canadian Bacon, 156
  Barbecued Beef 'n' Bean Burgers, 148
  Barbecued Limas and Beef, 155
  Barbecued Pinto Beans, 153
  Beef and Bulgur Chili Caliente, 26–27
  Black and White Chili with Pork, 30
  Blond Chili, 28
  Cannellini and Salmon Salad Toss, 150–151
  Corn 'n' Bean Chili, 29
  Easy Three-Bean Medley, 159
  Garden Vegetable-Beef Stew, 105
  Home-Style Barbecue Beef Wraps, 140
  Hominy and Beef Sausage Chili, 31
  Italian Sausage and Vegetable Chowder, 18–19
  Lamb and Black Bean Chili, 32
  Minestrone Stew, 25
  Picante Beef 'n' Beans, 157
  Smoked Sausage Chowder, 24
  Spiced Garbanzo Beans, 158
  Spicy Pintos on Tortillas, 152–153
  Taste-of-Italy Beans 'n' Sausage, 154
  Turkey Sausage Chili with Beans, 33
  Vegetarian Soybeans, 162
Beef
  Asparagus Cube Steak Roll-Ups, 107
  Barbecued Beef 'n' Bean Burgers, 148
  Barbecued Brisket 'n' Noodles, 99
  Barbecued Limas and Beef, 155
  Barley and Beef Stew, 163
  Beef and Bulgur Chili Caliente, 26–27
  Cabbage Burger Bake, 115
  Chile and Corn-Chip Meat Loaf, 109
  Chunky Spaghetti 'n' Turkey Meatballs, 82–83
  Confetti Meat Loaf, 110
  Corn 'n' Bean Chili, 29
  Creole Beef and Pepper Strips with Curly Noodles, 94–95
  Eight-Layer Casserole, 116
  Garden Vegetable-Beef Stew, 105
  Home-Style Barbecue Beef Wraps, 140
  Hominy and Beef Sausage Chili, 31
  Jicama-Cilantro Round Steak, 93
  Meatballs in Sun-Dried Tomato Gravy, 112–113
  Minestrone Stew, 25
  Moroccan-Style Pot Roast with Parsnips and Couscous, 101
  My Favorite Pasta Sauce, 81
  Navajo Beef and Chile Stew, 104
  New-Style Beef Stroganoff, 96
  Picante Beef 'n' Beans, 157
  Pot Roast with Avocado-Chile Topping, 100
  Pot Roast with Basil, Sun-Dried Tomatoes, and Pine Nuts, 102
  Sauerbraten-Style Short Ribs, 106
  Shortcut Chuck Roast with Mushroom Sauce, 103
  Sun-Dried Tomato Meat Loaf, 108
  Taste-of-Acapulco Flank Steak, 97
  Teriyaki Beef Pitas, 145
  Three-Pepper Steak, 98
Bell peppers
  Aloha Pork 'n' Rice, 127
  Barbecued Pinto Beans, 153
  Cantonese-Style Slow-Cooked Pork, 126
  Corn- and Turkey-Stuffed Bell Peppers, 177
  Creole Beef and Pepper Strips with Curly Noodles, 94–95
  Eight-Layer Casserole, 116
  Garden Vegetable-Beef Stew, 105
  Pasta with Easy Turkey-Vegetable Sauce, 80
  Pele's Hot Chicken Sandwich, 146–147
  Pesto- and Turkey-Stuffed Pita Pockets, 142–143
  Polynesian Pineapple Mango Relish, 202
  Rangoon Chicken Wraps, 138–139
  Roasted Red Pepper and Eggplant Soup, 11
  Three-Pepper Steak, 98
  Turkey Tostada Crisps, 75
  Vegetarian Soybeans, 162
Black and White Chili with Pork, 30
Black-Eyed Pea Soup, 20
Blond Chili, 28
Brandy
  Brandied Cherry Sauce, 200
  Brandied Fruit Compote, 201
Broccoli
  Cantonese-Style Slow-Cooked Pork, 126
  Pesto- and Turkey-Stuffed Pita Pockets, 142–143
  Steamed Broccoli-Corn Pudding, 180

Bulgur
Beef and Bulgur Chili Caliente, 26–27
Burgers
Barbecued Beef 'n' Bean Burgers, 148

Cabbage
Alsatian Pork Wraps, 141
Cabbage Burger Bake, 115
Chicken with Cabbage and Apples, 49
Italian Sausage and Vegetable Chowder, 18–19
Minestrone Stew, 25
Ragout of Red Cabbage with Port, 175
Vietnamese Pork in Savoy Cabbage, 128–129
Canadian bacon
Baked Beans with Canadian Bacon, 156
Sweet-and-Sour Squash, 176
Cannellini and Salmon Salad Toss, 150–151
Cantonese-Style Slow-Cooked Pork, 126
Capers
Sicilian Salsa, 168
Carrots
Barbecued Limas and Beef, 155
Barley and Beef Stew, 163
Black-Eyed Pea Soup, 20
Cabbage Burger Bake, 115
Cannellini and Salmon Salad Toss, 150–151
Cantonese-Style Slow-Cooked Pork, 126
Chicken with Fresh Herbs, 58
Chicken-Vegetable Pinwheels, 62
Confetti Meat Loaf, 110
Curried Lentils and Vegetables, 160–161
Garden Vegetable-Beef Stew, 105
Gingered Carrot Soup, 14
Gingered Carrots with Dijon Mustard, and Brown Sugar, 173
Hearty Confetti Fish Chowder, 22–23
My Favorite Pasta Sauce, 81
Rangoon Chicken Wraps, 138–139
Sunshine Carrot Pudding with Lemon Sauce, 190–191
Taco-Seasoned Turkey Pitas, 144
Cauliflower
Curried Cauliflower Appetizer, 169
Barbecued Beef 'n' Bean Burgers, 148

Barbecued Limas and Beef, 155
Barley and Beef Stew, 163
Chicken-Vegetable Pinwheels, 62
Classic Tomato-Vegetable Pasta Sauce, 179
Curried Lentils and Vegetables, 160–161
Potato- and Celery-Stuffed Chicken, 38–39
Sicilian Salsa, 168
Teriyaki Beef Pitas, 145
Wild Rice with Portobello Mushrooms, 166
Cereal
Pear Streusel, 199
Cheese
Blond Chili, 28
Fiesta Tamale Pie, 114
Greek Lamb, Vegetables, and Feta Cheese, 132–133
Pasta with Easy Turkey-Vegetable Sauce, 80
Pesto- and Turkey-Stuffed Pita Pockets, 142–143
Polenta-Chili Casserole, 63
Sorrento Potato and Cheese Packets, 172
South-of-the-Border Lasagna, 84
Spinach and Prosciutto Turkey Roulades, 72–73
Steamed Broccoli-Corn Pudding, 180
Turkey Tostada Crisps, 75
Cherries
Chunky Black Cherry Applesauce, 187
Dried Cherry and Apple Snack, 197
Cherry pie filling
Brandied Cherry Sauce, 200
Cherry tomatoes
Sorrento Potato and Cheese Packets, 172
Chicken
Chicken and Mango with Ginger-Curry Topping, 42–43
Chicken 'n' Vegetable Soup with Fresh Salsa, 16
Chicken-Vegetable Pinwheels, 62
Chicken with Cabbage and Apples, 49
Chicken with Fresh Herbs, 58
Chile-Citrus Chicken with Sun-Dried Tomatoes, 52
Cranberry-Orange Chicken, 50
Creamy Chicken 'n' Leeks, 59
Honey-Hoisin Chicken, 41
Old-fashioned Chicken 'n' Noodles, 44–45

Chicken (*continued*)
  Orange and Ginger Chicken, 48
  Peanut Butter 'n' Ginger Chicken, 51
  Peanutty Chicken 'n' Rice, 53
  Pele's Hot Chicken Sandwich,
    146–147
  Plum-Glazed Chicken, 46–47
  Polenta-Chili Casserole, 63
  Potato- and Celery-Stuffed Chicken,
    38–39
  Rangoon Chicken Wraps, 138–139
  Raspberried Drumsticks, 54
  Roasted Chicken Stuffed with Water
    Chestnuts and Bean Sprouts, 40
  Roasted Chicken with Rosemary and
    Garlic, 37
  Savory Chicken and Vegetables,
    60–61
  Spiced Chicken with Brown Rice,
    56–57
  Touch-of-the-Orient Chicken, 55
Chiles
  Barbecued Pinto Beans, 153
  Beef and Bulgur Chili Caliente,
    26–27
  Black-Eyed Pea Soup, 20
  Chile and Corn-Chip Meat Loaf, 109
  Chile-Citrus Chicken with Sun-Dried
    Tomatoes, 52
  Corn 'n' Bean Chili, 29
  Eggplant & Squash Veggie Dip, 170
  Fresh Salsa, 16, 65
  Hominy and Beef Sausage Chili, 31
  Navajo Beef and Chile Stew, 104
  Pot Roast with Avocado-Chile Top-
    ping, 100
  Spiced Garbanzo Beans, 158
  Spicy Pintos on Tortillas, 152–153
  Spicy Eggplant with Pine Nuts, 174
  Summer Vegetable Medley, 171
  Turkey Sausage Chili with Beans, 33
  Turkey Tortilla Soup, 17
  Turkey Tostada Crisps, 75
  Vegetarian Soybeans, 162
Chili
  Beef and Bulgur Chili Caliente,
    26–27
  Black and White Chili with Pork, 30
  Blond Chili, 28
  Corn 'n' Bean Chili, 29
  Hominy and Beef Sausage Chili, 31
  Lamb and Black Bean Chili, 32
  Turkey Sausage Chili with Beans, 33
Chowders
  Hearty Confetti Fish Chowder,
    22–23
  Italian Sausage and Vegetable Chow-
    der, 18

  Smoked Sausage Chowder, 24
Chunky Black Cherry Applesauce,
  187
Chunky Spaghetti 'n' Turkey Meat-
  balls, 82–83
Chutney
  Ginger-Nectarine Chutney, 125
  Pork- and Chutney-Stuffed Onions,
    178
  Rangoon Chicken Wraps, 138–139
Cilantro
  Fresh Salsa, 65
  Jicama-Cilantro Round Steak, 93
  Malaysian Turkey Cutlets, 74
  Taste-of-Acapulco Flank Steak, 97
Classic Tomato-Vegetable Pasta Sauce,
  179
Coconut milk
  Rangoon Chicken Wraps, 138–139
Coconut, toasting, 127
Coconut
  Aloha Pork 'n' Rice, 127
  Pork- and Chutney-Stuffed Onions,
    178
Confetti Meat Loaf, 110
Corn chips
  Chile and Corn-Chip Meat Loaf, 109
Corn
  Chicken 'n' Vegetable Soup with
    Fresh Salsa, 16
  Chicken with Fresh Herbs, 58
  Corn 'n' Bean Chili, 29
  Corn- and Turkey-Stuffed Bell Pep-
    pers, 177
  Double-Corn Stew, 21
  Eight-Layer Casserole, 116
  Fiesta Tamale Pie, 114
  Home-Style Barbecue Beef Wraps,
    140
  Navajo Beef and Chile Stew, 104
  Smoked Sausage Chowder, 24
  Steamed Broccoli-Corn Pudding, 180
  Summer Vegetable Medley, 171
  Taste-of-Acapulco Flank Steak, 97
Cornish hens
  Cornish Hens with Fresh Salsa, 65
  Tuscan-Style Cornish Hens, 64
Cornmeal
  Fiesta Tamale Pie, 114
  Steamed Broccoli-Corn Pudding, 180
Country-Style Ribs with Ginger-Nectar-
  ine Chutney, 125
Couscous
  Moroccan-Style Pot Roast with Pars-
    nips and Couscous, 101
  Sun-Dried Tomato Meat Loaf, 108
Cracker bread
  Alsatian Pork Wraps, 141

Cranberries
    Brandied Fruit Compote, 201
    Cranberry-Orange Chicken, 50
    Poached Apples 'n' Cranberries, 198
    Slow-Cooker Baked Cranberry
        Apples, 196
    Steamed Cranberry Pudding with Or-
        ange Blossom Sauce, 192–193
Cranberry juice
    Poached Apples 'n' Cranberries, 198
Cranberry sauce
    Cranberry-Port Pork Roast, 119
Creamy Chicken 'n' Leeks, 59
Creole Beef and Pepper Strips with
    Curly Noodles, 94–95
Cucumber
    Easy Three-Bean Medley, 159
Currants
    Autumn Surprise Relish, 203
    Creamy Chicken 'n' Leeks, 59
Curry powder
    Chicken and Mango with Ginger-
        Curry Topping, 42–43
    Country-Style Ribs with Ginger-Nec-
        tarine Chutney, 125
    Curried Cauliflower Appetizer, 169
    Curried Lentil-Leek Soup, 15
    Curried Lentils and Vegetables,
        160–161

Dates
    Steamed Pumpkin-Date Pudding
        with Rum Sauce, 188–189
Dill
    Cannellini and Salmon Salad Toss,
        150–151
Dips
    Eggplant & Squash Veggie Dip, 170
Double-Corn Stew, 21
Dried Cherry and Apple Snack, 197
Dried mixed fruit
    Brandied Fruit Compote, 201
    Lamb Shanks with Sweet Potatoes
        and Dried Fruit, 134

Easy Three-Bean Medley, 159
Eggplants
    Eggplant & Squash Veggie Dip, 170
    Roasted Red Pepper and Eggplant
        Soup, 11
    Sicilian Salsa, 168
    Spicy Eggplant with Pine Nuts, 174
Eight-Layer Casserole, 116
Enchilada sauce
    South-of-the-Border Lasagna, 84
    Turkey Porcupines in Enchilada
        Sauce, 90

Fat in the diet, percentage, 7
Fat (reducing amount in cooking), 2–3
Feast on Soups and Chili, 9–33
Fennel
    Cannellini and Salmon Salad Toss,
        150–151
    Fennel and Potato Soup, 13
Fiesta Tamale Pie, 114
Figs
    Garden of Eden Apples, 194–195
Fish
    Cannellini and Salmon Salad Toss,
        150–151
    Hearty Confetti Fish Chowder,
        22–23
Five-Spice Turkey Thighs, 76
Fragrant Brown Rice and Mushroom
    Soup, 10
Fresh Salsa, 16, 65
From the Garden to the Slow Cooker,
    167–183

Garden of Eden Apples, 194–195
Garden Vegetable-Beef Stew, 105
Garlic
    Garlic Lamb Dijon, 135
    Grace's Special Dolmas, 130–131
    Roasted Chicken with Rosemary and
        Garlic, 37
    Sicilian Salsa, 168
    Spiced Garbanzo Beans, 158
    Vietnamese Pork in Savoy Cabbage,
        128–129
Ginger
    Aloha Pork 'n' Rice, 127
    Autumn Surprise Relish, 203
    Chicken and Mango with Ginger-
        Curry Topping, 42–43
    Cranberry-Port Pork Roast, 119
    Gingered Carrot Soup, 14
    Ginger-Nectarine Chutney, 125
    Gingered Carrots with Dijon Mus-
        tard, and Brown Sugar, 173
    Honey-Hoisin Chicken, 41
    Jicama-Ginger Salsa, 68–69
    Orange and Ginger Chicken, 48
    Peanut Butter 'n' Ginger Chicken, 51
    Polynesian Pineapple Mango Relish,
        202
    Rhubarb-Apple Compote, 186
    Spiced Garbanzo Beans, 158
    Sunshine Carrot Pudding with
        Lemon Sauce, 190–191
    Vietnamese Pork in Savoy Cabbage,
        128–129
Gingersnaps
    Sauerbraten-Style Short Ribs, 106
Gold 'n' Green Squash Soup, 12

Golden Delicious Apples and Yam Scallop, 183
Good Eating with Wraps and Sandwiches, 137–148
Grace's Special Dolmas, 130–131
Grape leaves
 Grace's Special Dolmas, 130–131
 Stuffed Grape Leaves, 164–165
Greek Lamb, Vegetables, and Feta Cheese, 132–133

Ham
 Black-Eyed Pea Soup, 20
 Double-Corn Stew, 21
Harvest Pork Chops, 123
Healthful cooking in the slow cooker, 1–3
Hearty Confetti Fish Chowder, 22–23
Home-Style Barbecue Beef Wraps, 140
Hominy
 Double-Corn Stew, 21
 Hominy and Beef Sausage Chili, 31
Honey
 Brandied Fruit Compote, 201
 Garden of Eden Apples, 194–195
 Honey-Hoisin Chicken, 41
 Steamed Cranberry Pudding with Orange Blossom Sauce, 192–193
Horseradish
 Barbecued Brisket 'n' Noodles, 99
 Mustardy Orange-Flavored Pork Dinner, 121
 Pork Chops with Minted Herb Relish, 122
 Pot Roast with Avocado-Chile Topping, 100
 Potato and Turnip Slices with Mustard and Horseradish, 182

Introducton, 1–7
Italian Sausage and Vegetable Chowder, 18–19

Jicama
 Jicama-Cilantro Round Steak, 93
 Jicama-Ginger Salsa, 68–69
 Pele's Hot Chicken Sandwich, 146–147
 Turkey Tostada Crisps, 75

Kale
 Sweet-and-Sour Squash, 176

Lamb
 Garlic Lamb Dijon, 135
 Grace's Special Dolmas, 130–131
 Greek Lamb, Vegetables, and Feta Cheese, 132–133

Lamb and Black Bean Chili, 32
Lamb Shanks with Sweet Potatoes and Dried Fruit, 134
Lasagna
 South-of-the-Border Lasagna, 84
Leeks
 Chicken with Fresh Herbs, 58
 Classic Tomato-Vegetable Pasta Sauce, 179
 Confetti Meat Loaf, 110
 Creamy Chicken 'n' Leeks, 59
 Curried Lentil-Leek Soup, 15
 Garden Vegetable-Beef Stew, 105
 Polenta-Chili Casserole, 63
 Summer Vegetable Medley, 171
 Tarragon-Mustard Turkey with Fettuccine, 78–79
Lemon
 Cranberry-Port Pork Roast, 119
 Lemon Sauce, 190–191
 Sauerbraten-Style Short Ribs, 106
Lentils
 Curried Lentil-Leek Soup, 15
 Curried Lentils and Vegetables, 160–161

Malaysian Turkey Cutlets, 74
Mangoes
 Chicken and Mango with Ginger-Curry Topping, 42–43
 Polynesian Pineapple Mango Relish, 202
Mayonnaise
 Curried Cauliflower Appetizer, 169
Meat loaf
 Chile and Corn-Chip Meat Loaf, 109
 Confetti Meat Loaf, 110
 Sun-Dried Tomato Meat Loaf, 108
Meatballs
 Chunky Spaghetti 'n' Turkey Meatballs, 82–83
 Meatballs in Sun-Dried Tomato Gravy, 112–113
 Porcupine Meatballs in Tomato Sauce, 111
 Raspberry-Glazed Turkey Meatballs, 88–89
 Turkey Porcupines in Enchilada Sauce, 90
Minestrone Stew, 25
Mint
 Malaysian Turkey Cutlets, 74
 Pork Chops with Minted Herb Relish, 122
 Vietnamese Pork in Savoy Cabbage, 128–129

Mixed vegetables
  Savory Chicken and Vegetables,
    60–61
Molasses
  Baked Beans with Canadian Bacon,
    156
  Barbecued Pinto Beans, 153
  Home-Style Barbecue Beef Wraps,
    140
Mushroom soup
  Chicken 'n' Vegetable Soup with
    Fresh Salsa, 16
  Classic Tomato-Vegetable Pasta
    Sauce, 179
  Fragrant Brown Rice and Mushroom
    Soup, 10
  New-Style Beef Stroganoff, 96
  Pele's Hot Chicken Sandwich,
    146–147
  Savory Chicken and Vegetables,
    60–61
  Shortcut Chuck Roast with Mush-
    room Sauce, 103
  Three-Pepper Steak, 98
  Wild Rice with Portobello Mush-
    rooms, 166
Mustard
  Alsatian Pork Wraps, 141
  Baked Beans with Canadian Bacon,
    156
  Barbecued Brisket 'n' Noodles, 99
  Barbecued Limas and Beef, 155
  Cranberry-Orange Chicken, 50
  Garlic Lamb Dijon, 135
  Gingered Carrots with Dijon Mus-
    tard, and Brown Sugar, 173
  Home-Style Barbecue Beef Wraps, 140
  Mustardy Orange-Flavored Pork Din-
    ner, 121
  Pork Chops with Minted Herb Relish,
    122
  Potato and Turnip Slices with Mus-
    tard and Horseradish, 182
  Raspberried Drumsticks, 54
  Tarragon-Mustard Turkey with Fet-
    tuccine, 78–79
My Favorite Pasta Sauce, 81

Navajo Beef and Chile Stew, 104
Nectarines
  Ginger-Nectarine Chutney, 125
New-Style Beef Stroganoff, 96
Noodles
  Barbecued Brisket 'n' Noodles, 99
  Creole Beef and Pepper Strips with
    Curly Noodles, 94–95
  Old-fashioned Chicken 'n' Noodles,
    44–45

South-of-the-Border Lasagna, 84
Nutritional Analysis, 7

Oats
  Dried Cherry and Apple Snack, 197
  Raspberry-Glazed Turkey Meatballs,
    88–89
Old-fashioned Chicken 'n' Noodles,
    44–45
Olives
  Sicilian Salsa, 168
Onion soup mix
  Shortcut Chuck Roast with Mush-
    room Sauce, 103
Onions
  Baked Beans with Canadian Bacon,
    156
  Baked Onions and Apples with Cinna-
    mon, 181
  Barbecued Limas and Beef, 155
  Barbecued Pinto Beans, 153
  Barley and Beef Stew, 163
  Beef and Bulgur Chili Caliente,
    26–27
  Black and White Chili with Pork, 30
  Cannellini and Salmon Salad Toss,
    150–151
  Cantonese-Style Slow-Cooked Pork,
    126
  Corn 'n' Bean Chili, 29
  Corn- and Turkey-Stuffed Bell Pep-
    pers, 177
  Curried Lentils and Vegetables,
    160–161
  Eggplant & Squash Veggie Dip, 170
  Grace's Special Dolmas, 130–131
  Hominy and Beef Sausage Chili, 31
  Lamb and Black Bean Chili, 32
  Mustardy Orange-Flavored Pork Din-
    ner, 121
  Navajo Beef and Chile Stew, 104
  Picante Beef 'n' Beans, 157
  Polynesian Pineapple Mango Relish,
    202
  Pork and Apple Hot-Pot, 120
  Pork with Sweet Potatoes, Apples,
    and Sauerkraut, 124
  Pork- and Chutney-Stuffed Onions,
    178
  Ragout of Red Cabbage with Port,
    175
  Sauerbraten-Style Short Ribs, 106
  Sicilian Salsa, 168
  Sorrento Potato and Cheese Packets,
    172
  Spiced Garbanzo Beans, 158
  Spicy Eggplant with Pine Nuts, 174
  Spicy Pintos on Tortillas, 152–153

Onions (*continued*)
   Teriyaki Beef Pitas, 145
   Vegetarian Soybeans, 162
   Wild Rice with Portobello Mushrooms, 166
Orange juice
   Chile-Citrus Chicken with Sun-Dried Tomatoes, 52
   Cranberry-Orange Chicken, 50
   Lamb Shanks with Sweet Potatoes and Dried Fruit, 134
   Mustardy Orange-Flavored Pork Dinner, 121
   Orange and Ginger Chicken, 48
   Orange Blossom Sauce, 192–193
   Spiced Chicken with Brown Rice, 56–57
Orange peel
   Ragout of Red Cabbage with Port, 175
   Rhubarb-Apple Compote, 186
Oranges
   Autumn Surprise Relish, 203
   Brandied Fruit Compote, 201
   Gold 'n' Green Squash Soup, 12
   Harvest Pork Chops, 123

Parsley
   Pesto- and Turkey-Stuffed Pita Pockets, 142–143
Parsnips
   Moroccan-Style Pot Roast with Parsnips and Couscous, 101
Pasta sauce
   Classic Tomato-Vegetable Pasta Sauce, 179
Pasta
   Chunky Spaghetti 'n' Turkey Meatballs, 82–83
   Italian Sausage and Vegetable Chowder, 18–19
   Minestrone Stew, 25
   Pasta with Easy Turkey-Vegetable Sauce, 80
   Tarragon-Mustard Turkey with Fettuccine, 78–79
Peanut butter
   Aloha Pork 'n' Rice, 127
   Peanut Butter 'n' Ginger Chicken, 51
   Rangoon Chicken Wraps, 138–139
   Tijuana Turkey, 70–71
Peanuts
   Peanutty Chicken 'n' Rice, 53
Pear Streusel, 199
Peas
   Curried Lentils and Vegetables, 160–161

Pecans
   Country-Style Ribs with Ginger-Nectarine Chutney, 125
   Golden Delicious Apples and Yam Scallop, 183
Pele's Hot Chicken Sandwich, 146–147
Pesto- and Turkey-Stuffed Pita Pockets, 142–143
Picante Beef 'n' Beans, 157
Picante sauce
   Easy Three-Bean Medley, 159
   Picante Beef 'n' Beans, 157
   Smoked Sausage Chowder, 24
Pimientos
   Hearty Confetti Fish Chowder, 22–23
Pine nuts, toasting, 165
Pine nuts
   Pot Roast with Basil, Sun-Dried Tomatoes, and Pine Nuts, 102
   Sicilian Salsa, 168
   Spicy Eggplant with Pine Nuts, 174
   Spinach and Prosciutto Turkey Roulades, 72–73
   Stuffed Grape Leaves, 164–165
Pineapple juice
   Pele's Hot Chicken Sandwich, 146–147
Pineapple
   Brandied Fruit Compote, 201
   Polynesian Pineapple Mango Relish, 202
   Sunshine Carrot Pudding with Lemon Sauce, 190–191
Pita bread
   Eggplant & Squash Veggie Dip, 170
   Pesto- and Turkey-Stuffed Pita Pockets, 142–143
   Taco-Seasoned Turkey Pitas, 144
   Teriyaki Beef Pitas, 145
Plum preserves
   Plum-Glazed Chicken, 46–47
Poached Apples 'n' Cranberries, 198
Polenta-Chili Casserole, 63
Polynesian Pineapple Mango Relish, 202
Porcupine Meatballs in Tomato Sauce, 111
Pork
   Aloha Pork 'n' Rice, 127
   Alsatian Pork Wraps, 141
   Black and White Chili with Pork, 30
   Cantonese-Style Slow-Cooked Pork, 126
   Confetti Meat Loaf, 110
   Country-Style Ribs with Ginger-Nectarine Chutney, 125
   Cranberry-Port Pork Roast, 119
   Harvest Pork Chops, 123

Mustardy Orange-Flavored Pork Dinner, 121
Pork and Apple Hot-Pot, 120
Pork Chops with Minted Herb Relish, 122
Pork with Sweet Potatoes, Apples, and Sauerkraut, 124
Pork- and Chutney-Stuffed Onions, 178
Vietnamese Pork in Savoy Cabbage, 128–129
Wild Rice with Portobello Mushrooms, 166
Pot Roast with Avocado-Chile Topping, 100
Pot Roast with Basil, Sun-Dried Tomatoes, and Pine Nuts, 102
Potatoes
Alsatian Pork Wraps, 141
Asparagus Cube Steak Roll-Ups, 107
Chicken 'n' Vegetable Soup with Fresh Salsa, 16
Fennel and Potato Soup, 13
Garden Vegetable-Beef Stew, 105
Hearty Confetti Fish Chowder, 22–23
Potato and Turnip Slices with Mustard and Horseradish, 182
Potato- and Celery-Stuffed Chicken, 38–39
Savory Chicken and Vegetables, 60–61
Sorrento Potato and Cheese Packets, 172
Prosciutto
Spinach and Prosciutto Turkey Roulades, 72–73
Tuscan-Style Cornish Hens, 64
Puddings
Almond Bread Pudding with Brandied Cherry Sauce, 200
Steamed Cranberry Pudding with Orange Blossom Sauce, 192–193
Steamed Pumpkin-Date Pudding with Rum Sauce, 188–189
Sunshine Carrot Pudding with Lemon Sauce, 190–191
Pumpkin
Steamed Pumpkin-Date Pudding with Rum Sauce, 188–189

Ragout of Red Cabbage with Port, 175
Raisins
Brandied Fruit Compote, 201
Country-Style Ribs with Ginger-Nectarine Chutney, 125
Cranberry-Port Pork Roast, 119
Polynesian Pineapple Mango Relish, 202

Sunshine Carrot Pudding with Lemon Sauce, 190–191
Rangoon Chicken Wraps, 138–139
Raspberry fruit spread
Raspberried Drumsticks, 54
Raspberry-Glazed Turkey Meatballs, 88–89
Relish
Autumn Surprise Relish, 203
Polynesian Pineapple Mango Relish, 202
Rhubarb-Apple Compote, 186
Rice
Aloha Pork 'n' Rice, 127
Rice
Cabbage Burger Bake, 115
Eight-Layer Casserole, 116
Fragrant Brown Rice and Mushroom Soup, 10
Grace's Special Dolmas, 130–131
Peanutty Chicken 'n' Rice, 53
Porcupine Meatballs in Tomato Sauce, 111
Rangoon Chicken Wraps, 138–139
Round Sesame Turkey Loaf, 86
Spiced Chicken with Brown Rice, 56–57
Stuffed Grape Leaves, 164–165
Tijuana Turkey, 70–71
Turkey Porcupines in Enchilada Sauce, 90
Wild Rice with Portobello Mushrooms, 166
Roasted Chicken Stuffed with Water Chestnuts and Bean Sprouts, 40
Roasted Chicken with Rosemary and Garlic, 37
Roasted Red Pepper and Eggplant Soup, 11
Rosemary
Garlic Lamb Dijon, 135
Roasted Chicken with Rosemary and Garlic, 37
Sorrento Potato and Cheese Packets, 172
Round Sesame Turkey Loaf, 86
Rum Sauce, 188–189

Sage
Taste-of-Italy Beans 'n' Sausage, 154
Tuscan-Style Cornish Hens, 64
Salad
Cannellini and Salmon Salad Toss, 150–151
Salmon
Cannellini and Salmon Salad Toss, 150–151

Salsa
  Fiesta Tamale Pie, 114
  Fresh Salsa, 16, 65
  Jicama-Ginger Salsa, 68–69
  Sicilian Salsa, 168
  Taste-of-the-Southwest Turkey Loaf, 85
Satisfying Tastes with Pork and Lamb, 117–135
Sauces
  Brandied Cherry Sauce, 200
  Lemon Sauce, 190–191
  My Favorite Pasta Sauce, 81
  Orange Blossom Sauce, 192–193
  Rum Sauce, 188–189
Sauerbraten-Style Short Ribs, 106
Sauerkraut
  Pork with Sweet Potatoes, Apples, and Sauerkraut, 124
Savory Chicken and Vegetables, 60–61
Sesame seeds, toasting, 55
Sesame seeds
  Five-Spice Turkey Thighs, 76
  Honey-Hoisin Chicken, 41
  Round Sesame Turkey Loaf, 86
  Touch-of-the-Orient Chicken, 55
Shortcut Chuck Roast with Mushroom Sauce, 103
Sicilian Salsa, 168
Slow-and-Easy Beans and Grains, 149–166
Slow-Cooker Baked Cranberry Apples, 196
Slow-Cooking Turkey Discoveries, 67–90
Smoked Sausage Chowder, 24
Sodium, reducing, 7
Sorrento Potato and Cheese Packets, 172
Soups
  Black-Eyed Pea Soup, 20
  Chicken 'n' Vegetable Soup with Fresh Salsa, 16
  Curried Lentil-Leek Soup, 15
  Fennel and Potato Soup, 13
  Fragrant Brown Rice and Mushroom Soup, 10
  Gingered Carrot Soup, 14
  Gold 'n' Green Squash Soup, 12
  Roasted Red Pepper and Eggplant Soup, 11
  Turkey Tortilla Soup, 17
Sour cream
  Garden of Eden Apples, 194–195
  New-Style Beef Stroganoff, 96
  Poached Apples 'n' Cranberries, 198
South-of-the-Border Lasagna, 84

Soy sauce
  Touch-of-the-Orient Chicken, 55
  Vietnamese Pork in Savoy Cabbage, 128–129
  Wild Rice with Portobello Mushrooms, 166
Spaghetti
  Chunky Spaghetti 'n' Turkey Meatballs, 82–83
  Classic Tomato-Vegetable Pasta Sauce, 179
Spaghetti sauce
  Cabbage Burger Bake, 115
Spiced Chicken with Brown Rice, 56–57
Spiced Garbanzo Beans, 158
Spicy Eggplant with Pine Nuts, 174
Spicy Pintos on Tortillas, 152–153
Spinach
  Spinach and Prosciutto Turkey Roulades, 72–73
  Taco-Seasoned Turkey Pitas, 144
Squash (see also Zucchini)
  Autumn Surprise Relish, 203
  Eggplant & Squash Veggie Dip, 170
  Gold 'n' Green Squash Soup, 12
  Greek Lamb, Vegetables, and Feta Cheese, 132–133
  Harvest Pork Chops, 123
  Italian Sausage and Vegetable Chowder, 18–19
  Sweet-and-Sour Squash, 176
  Teriyaki Turkey Loaf, 87
Steamed Broccoli-Corn Pudding, 180
Steamed Cranberry Pudding with Orange Blossom Sauce, 192–193
Steamed Pumpkin-Date Pudding with Rum Sauce, 188–189
Stews
  Barley and Beef Stew, 163
  Double-Corn Stew, 21
  Garden Vegetable-Beef Stew, 105
  Minestrone Stew, 25
  Navajo Beef and Chile Stew, 104
  Turkey, Yam, and Apple Stew, 77
Stroganoff
  New-Style Beef Stroganoff, 96
Stuffed Grape Leaves, 164–165
Summer Vegetable Medley, 171
Sun-Dried Tomato Meat Loaf, 108
Sunshine Carrot Pudding with Lemon Sauce, 190–191
Sweet potatoes (see also Yams)
  Lamb Shanks with Sweet Potatoes and Dried Fruit, 134
  Mustardy Orange-Flavored Pork Dinner, 121
  Pork with Sweet Potatoes, Apples, and Sauerkraut, 124

Sweet-and-sour sauce
  Sweet-and-Sour Squash, 176

Taco-Seasoned Turkey Pitas, 144
Tarragon-Mustard Turkey with Fettuc-
  cine, 78–79
Taste-of-Acapulco Flank Steak, 97
Taste-of-Italy Beans 'n' Sausage, 154
Taste-of-the-Southwest Turkey Loaf,
  85
Teriyaki Beef Pitas, 145
Teriyaki Turkey Loaf, 87
Three-Pepper Steak, 98
Tijuana Turkey, 70–71
Tomatillos
  South-of-the-Border Lasagna, 84
  Taste-of-Acapulco Flank Steak, 97
Tomato paste
  Barbecued Limas and Beef, 155
  Sicilian Salsa, 168
Tomato puree
  Classic Tomato-Vegetable Pasta
    Sauce, 179
Tomato sauce
  Barbecued Beef 'n' Bean Burgers,
    148
  Eight-Layer Casserole, 116
  Porcupine Meatballs in Tomato
    Sauce, 111
  Touch-of-the-Orient Chicken, 55
Tomatoes
  Beef and Bulgur Chili Caliente,
    26–27
  Chicken with Fresh Herbs, 58
  Corn- and Turkey-Stuffed Bell Pep-
    pers, 177
  Creole Beef and Pepper Strips with
    Curly Noodles, 94–95
  Double-Corn Stew, 21
  Easy Three-Bean Medley, 159
  Fresh Salsa, 16, 65
  Italian Sausage and Vegetable Chow-
    der, 18–19
  Jicama-Cilantro Round Steak, 93
  Jicama-Ginger Salsa, 68–69
  Lamb and Black Bean Chili, 32
  Minestrone Stew, 25
  My Favorite Pasta Sauce, 81
  Navajo Beef and Chile Stew, 104
  Pasta with Easy Turkey-Vegetable
    Sauce, 80
  Picante Beef 'n' Beans, 157
  Pork Chops with Minted Herb Relish,
    122
  Spiced Garbanzo Beans, 158
  Spicy Eggplant with Pine Nuts, 174
  Summer Vegetable Medley, 171
  Taste-of-Italy Beans 'n' Sausage, 154

Turkey Sausage Chili with Beans, 33
Turkey Tortilla Soup, 17
Vegetarian Soybeans, 162
Tomatoes, dried
  Blond Chili, 28
  Chile-Citrus Chicken with Sun-Dried
    Tomatoes, 52
  Meatballs in Sun-Dried Tomato
    Gravy, 112–113
  Pot Roast with Basil, Sun-Dried To-
    matoes, and Pine Nuts, 102
  Sun-Dried Tomato Meat Loaf, 108
Tortillas
  Easy Three-Bean Medley, 159
  Home-Style Barbecue Beef Wraps,
    140
  Rangoon Chicken Wraps, 138–139
  Spicy Pintos on Tortillas, 152–153
  Turkey Tortilla Soup, 17
  Turkey Tostada Crisps, 75
Touch-of-the-Orient Chicken, 55
Turkey (see also Turkey sausage)
  Five-Spice Turkey Thighs, 76
  Malaysian Turkey Cutlets, 74
  My Favorite Pasta Sauce, 81
  Pasta with Easy Turkey-Vegetable
    Sauce, 80
  Pesto- and Turkey-Stuffed Pita Pock-
    ets, 142–143
  Polenta-Chili Casserole, 63
  Raspberry-Glazed Turkey Meatballs,
    88–89
  Round Sesame Turkey Loaf, 86
  Spinach and Prosciutto Turkey Rou-
    lades, 72–73
  Taco-Seasoned Turkey Pitas, 144
  Taste-of-the-Southwest Turkey Loaf,
    85
  Teriyaki Turkey Loaf, 87
  Tijuana Turkey, 70–71
  Turkey Porcupines in Enchilada
    Sauce, 90
  Turkey Tostada Crisps, 75
  Turkey with Jicama-Ginger Salsa,
    68–69
  Turkey Tortilla Soup, 17
  Turkey, Yam, and Apple Stew, 77
Turkey sausage
  Blond Chili, 28
  Chicken-Vegetable Pinwheels, 62
  Chunky Spaghetti 'n' Turkey Meat-
    balls, 82–83
  Corn- and Turkey-Stuffed Bell Pep-
    pers, 177
  Italian Sausage and Vegetable Chow-
    der, 18–19
  Meatballs in Sun-Dried Tomato
    Gravy, 112–113

Turkey sausage (*continued*)
Smoked Sausage Chowder, 24
South-of-the-Border Lasagna, 84
Taste-of-Italy Beans 'n' Sausage, 154
Turkey Sausage Chili with Beans, 33
Turnips
Barley and Beef Stew, 163
Potato and Turnip Slices with Mustard and Horseradish, 182
Tuscan-Style Cornish Hens, 64

Using a slow cooker, 3–6

Vegetable juice
Vegetarian Soybeans, 162
Vegetarian Soybeans, 162
Vietnamese Pork in Savoy Cabbage, 128–129

Walnuts
Slow-Cooker Baked Cranberry Apples, 196
Orange and Ginger Chicken, 48
Roasted Chicken Stuffed with Water Chestnuts and Bean Sprouts, 40
Round Sesame Turkey Loaf, 86
Teriyaki Turkey Loaf, 87
Vietnamese Pork in Savoy Cabbage, 128–129
Welcome Ways with Beef, 91–116
Why use a slow cooker?, 6

Wild Rice with Portobello Mushrooms, 166
Wraps
Alsatian Pork Wraps, 141
Home-Style Barbecue Beef Wraps, 140
Rangoon Chicken Wraps, 138–139

Yams (see also Sweet potatoes)
Curried Lentils and Vegetables, 160–161
Golden Delicious Apples and Yam Scallop, 183
Turkey, Yam, and Apple Stew, 77
Year-Round Desserts and Accompaniments, 185–203
Yogurt
Curried Cauliflower Appetizer, 169
Curried Lentils and Vegetables, 160–161
Spiced Chicken with Brown Rice, 56–57

Zucchini
Confetti Meat Loaf, 110
Pele's Hot Chicken Sandwich, 146–147
Summer Vegetable Medley, 171
Taste-of-the-Southwest Turkey Loaf, 85
Vegetarian Soybeans, 162